The LWW MRI Teaching File Series

MRI of the Brain II

Second Edition

The LWW MRI Teaching File Series

SERIES EDITORS

Robert B. Lufkin
William G. Bradley, Jr.
Michael Brant-Zawadzki

MRI of the Brain I

William G. Bradley, Jr., Michael Brant-Zawadzki, and Jane Cambray-Forker

MRI of the Brain II

Michael Brant-Zawadzki, Jane Cambray-Forker, and William G. Bradley, Jr.

MRI of the Spine

Jeffrey S. Ross

MRI of the Head and Neck

Robert B. Lufkin, Alexandra Borges, Kim N. Nguyen, and Yoshimi Anzai

MRI of the Musculoskeletal System

Karence K. Chan and Mini Pathria

Pediatric MRI

Rosalind B. Dietrich

The LWW MRI Teaching File Series

MRI of the Brain II

Second Edition

Editors

Michael Brant-Zawadzki, M.D.
Medical Director
Department of Radiology
Hoag Memorial Hospital Presbyterian
Newport Beach, California

Clinical Professor of Diagnostic Radiology
Stanford University
Stanford, California

William G. Bradley, Jr., M.D., Ph.D.
Director, MRI and Radiology Research
Department of Radiology
Long Beach Memorial Medical Center
Long Beach, California

Professor
Department of Radiological Sciences
University of California, Irvine
Orange, California

Jane Cambray-Forker, D.O.
Director, Spinal Imaging
Department of Radiology
St. Joseph's Hospital
Orange, California

Assistant Clinical Professor
Department of Diagnostic Radiology
University of California, Irvine
College of Medicine
Orange, California

Associate Editors

Peter Brotchie, M.B.B.S., Ph.D.
Director of MRI
The Geelong Hospital
Geelong, Victoria, Australia

Sattam Saud Lingawi, M.D.
The University Hospital
King Abdulaziz University
Jeddah, Saudi Arabia

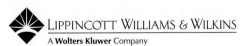
LIPPINCOTT WILLIAMS & WILKINS
A Wolters Kluwer Company
Philadelphia · Baltimore · New York · London
Buenos Aires · Hong Kong · Sydney · Tokyo

Acquisitions Editor: Joyce-Rachel John
Developmental Editor: Denise Martin
Production Editor: W. Christopher Granville
Manufacturing Manager: Tim Reynolds
Cover Designer: Jeane Norton
Compositor: Maryland Composition
Printer: Maple Press

© 2001 by LIPPINCOTT WILLIAMS & WILKINS
530 Walnut Street
Philadelphia, PA 19106-3780 USA
LWW. com

Printed in the USA

Library of Congress Cataloging-in-Publication Data

MRI of the Brain I / editors, William G. Bradley, Jr., Michael Brant-Zawadzki, Jane Cambray-Forker; associate editors, Peter Brotchie, Sattam Saud Lingawi.— 2nd ed.
    p. ; cm. — (The LWW MRI teaching file series)
  Rev. ed. of: MRI of the brain. New York : Raven Press, c1991.
  Includes bibliographical references and index.
  ISBN 0-7817-2569-0 (Volume 1)
  ISBN 0-7817-2568-2 (Volume 2)
    1. Brain—Magnetic resonance imaging. 2. Brain—Diseases—Diagnosis. I. Bradley, William G. II. Brant-Zawadzki, Michael. III. Cambray-Forker, Jane. IV. MRI of the brain. V. Series.
    [DNLM: 1. Brain Diseases—diagnosis. 2. Magnetic Resonance Imaging. WL 348 B8128 2000]
RC386.6.M34 B74 2000
616.8'047548–dc21

                                             00-061099

10 9 8 7 6 5 4 3 2 1

Although we do not want to take anything away
from our wives, children, mentors, or students,
this volume is dedicated to the neurosis which
results in our writing books when
we could be playing golf or going fishing.

W. G. B.
M. B.-Z.

To my husband, Gerry, for his unwavering support, encouragement, and faith in me.
To my children, Britton and Shane, who make everything worthwhile.
To my teachers, mentors, and friends,
Drs. Michael Huckman, Glenn Geremia, and William Greenlee.

I would like to give special thanks to Robyn Francis for all her hard work—
I couldn't have done it without you!
Thank you to Dr. Michael Brant-Zawadzki for your help, guidance, and support.
Thanks to all at Irvine Imaging Services.

J. C.-F.

CONTENTS

Note: Unless otherwise indicated, all cases have been submitted by Jane Cambray-Forker, D.O. and Michael Brant-Zawadzki, M.D., Hoag Memorial Hospital, Newport Beach, California.

PREFACE

Twelve years ago, we approached Mary Rogers, then the president of Raven Press (now Lippincott Williams & Wilkins) to do a 1,000-case, 10-volume MR Teaching File. The fact that they have asked us to do it again means it must have been successful. This volume is one of two volumes on the brain and again is edited by us with major contributions from Drs. Cambray, Lingawi, and Brotchie. To preserve the concept of a teaching file, the cases are essentially in randrom order without grouping by category. This allows the reader to first view the images and read the clinical history followed by the diagnosis and discussion. The discussion has been kept intentionally brief to allow coverage of multiple cases in a short period of time. References are provided for additional reading. As the reader will see, the latest in MR technology—echo planar diffusion, echo planar perfusion, and spectroscopy—are included in this volume. Comparison with the first edition published 10 years ago gives even the most casual observer a good concept of how far we have come in the clinical application of MRI technology. We hope you enjoy reading this teaching file as much as we enjoyed putting it together.

A few people deserve special thanks for this volume including the 1999–2000 MR Fellows at Long Beach Memorial Medical Center, Dr. Sandy Patel (MR Fellow 1997–98), and several residents from the University of California at Irvine who rotated through during the year. Dr. Cambray-Forker at Hoag Memorial Hospital was the major force behind almost all of the content contributed from Hoag and Robyn Francis was an invaluable assistant. We would also like to thank Jim Ryan at Lippincott Williams & Wilkins who persisted in his efforts to put together this second edition and Joyce-Rachel John whose persistence resulted in our completing this project in a timely fashion.

William G. Bradley, Jr., M.D., Ph.D.
Michael Brant-Zawadzki, M.D.

MRI of the Brain II

Second Edition

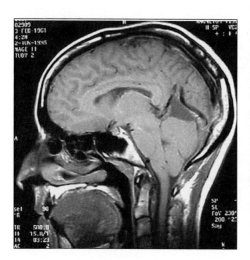

FIGURE 1.1A

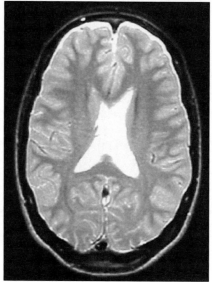

FIGURE 1.1B

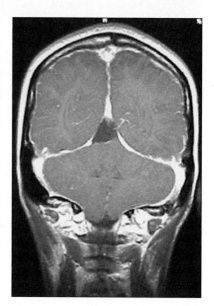

FIGURE 1.1C

CLINICAL HISTORY

A 34-year-old female with 3-month history of headaches associated with a sensation of "hearing her own voice."

FINDINGS

Sagittal T1-weighted acquisition (Fig. 1.1A) demonstrates cerebellar tonsillar ectopia below the level of the foramen magnum. There is downward displacement of the fourth ventricle with exaggeration of the superior cerebellar cistern, creating a sagging posterior fossa appearance. Axial T2-weighted acquisition (Fig. 1.1B) shows high signal in the extraaxial space anterior to the frontal lobes extending into the interhemispheric region. Following intravenous contrast (Fig. 1.1C), coronal T1-weighted images demonstrate diffuse, thick enhancement of the pachymeninges, including the tentorium and falx cerebri. Again note the downward displacement of the cerebellar tonsils.

DIAGNOSIS

Intracranial hypotension.

DISCUSSION

Spontaneous intracranial hypotension (SIH) is a syndrome similar to that which occurs following lumbar puncture. In this entity, however, there is usually no history of surgical intervention, significant trauma, or lumbar puncture. It is presumed to be the result of minor head or back trauma with subsequent tear of the arachnoid membrane surrounding a nerve root, which results in the continuous leakage of cerebrospinal fluid (CSF). The actual location of the CSF leak usually cannot be identified. With the progressive loss of fluid, the CSF pressure drops. In most cases, the CSF pressure is extremely low (less than 30 mm of water). Often a pressure cannot be obtained at lumbar puncture; this is known as a "dry tap."

The syndrome is characterized clinically by severe postural headache. Symptoms are aggravated by sitting upright or standing and are relieved by lying down. Cranial neuropathies, nausea, vomiting, stiff neck, and diplopia are less common presenting complaints. The duration is usually brief; however, symptoms can persist for months or even years. Symptoms usually regress spontaneously.

Diffuse pachymeningeal thickening and enhancement is the primary radiographic finding. It is typically described as linear and symmetric, involving both the supra- and infratentorial dura. The leptomeninges are not involved and therefore there is no involvement of the depths of the cortical sulci, the Sylvian fissures, or the brainstem surface. The cause of this dural enhancement is thought to be vascular dilatation (compensating for loss of CSF volume) as opposed to meningeal inflammation. The low CSF pressure can also result in brain "settling" and thus inferior displacement of the cerebellar tonsils through the foramen magnum, mimicking a Chiari I malformation (as seen in this case), and obliteration of the suprasellar cistern. It is the consequent traction on the exiting cranial nerves that produces the neuropathies associated with SIH syndrome. It has been postulated that downward herniation of the posterior fossa would be more frequently seen on MRI in SIH patients if they were scanned in the upright position. Tonsillar herniation in SIH is reversible when the syndrome resolves. Secondary findings in SIH include subdural hematoma and/or hygroma. This is presumably the result of the cortex pulling away from the inner table of the calvarium with the precipitous drop in CSF pressure and volume, causing tearing of the bridging cortical veins. Slitlike ventricles, small basal cisterns, and Sylvian fissures have also been described. A reported spinal manifestation of SIH is ventral extradural fluid collections directly related to the CSF leak. Although nonspecific, this finding can help in the diagnosis of SIH in the presence of classic intracranial findings. Additionally, the location of the fluid collection within the spinal canal can help determine the level of the CSF leak. Although generally of low diagnostic yield, cisternography can be used to detect CSF leak in cases of SIH. Accumulation of tracer within the spinal extraarachnoid space is suggestive of leak. Early bladder visualization during cisternography is also a sign of CSF leak due to the rapid systemic absorption of radionuclide.

Initial treatment of SIH headache is with bedrest, analgesics, caffeine, and steroids. If there is no improvement, intravenous or oral caffeine may be of benefit. If the patient continues to be symptomatic, a blood patch is indicated.

The intracranial imaging findings in SIH are usually dramatic but nonspecific. Other etiologies for diffuse pachymeningeal enhancement include inflammatory and neoplastic disease. In these entities, however, the dural enhancement is more irregular and nodular in appearance.

SUGGESTED READINGS

Fishman RA, Dillon WP. Dural enhancement and cerebral displacement secondary to intracranial hypotension. *Neurology* 1993;43:609–611.

Mokri B, Peipgras DG, Miller GM. Syndrome of orthostatic headaches and diffuse pachymeningeal gadolinium enhancement. *Mayo Clin Proc* 1997;72:400–413.

O'Carroll CP, Brant-Zawadzki MN. The syndrome of spontaneous intracranial hypotension. *Cephalalgia* 1999;19:80–86.

Rabin BM, Roychowdhury S, Meyer JR, et al. Spontaneous intracranial hypotension: spinal MR findings. *AJNR* 1998;19:1034–1039.

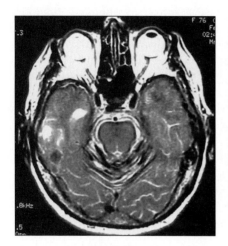

FIGURE 2.1A

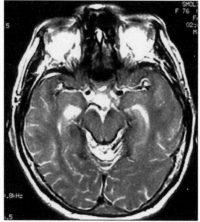

FIGURE 2.1B

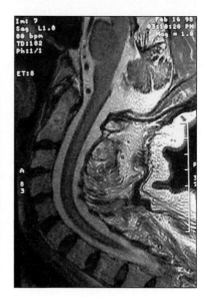

FIGURE 2.1C

CLINICAL HISTORY

A 76-year-old female with vertigo.

FINDINGS

Axial T2-weighted images (Fig. 2.1A,B) demonstrate curvilinear regions of very low signal coating the surface of the brain, pons, and tectal plate. Similar regions of low signal are also seen along the folia of the cerebellum. Sagittal T2-weighted acquisition through the craniovertebral junction and upper cervical spine (Fig. 2.1C) shows low-signal material coating the surface of the cervical spinal cord.

DIAGNOSIS

Superficial siderosis.

DISCUSSION

Dural malformations, neoplasms, and other vascular lesions that cause chronic recurrent subarachnoid hemorrhage can lead to deposition of hemosiderin within the central nervous system, known as superficial siderosis. Hemosiderin and reactive macrophages are deposited within the leptomeninges and subpial tissue. The brainstem, cerebellum, and cranial nerves coursing through the basal cisterns are most frequently affected. Siderosis has also been reported as a late complication of posterior fossa surgery.

Patients typically present with progressive hearing loss, cerebellar dysfunction, pyramidal tract signs, and, in its end stage, dementia. Cranial nerves II, V, VII, and VIII are commonly involved. The eighth cranial nerve is the most sensitive to the effects of hemosiderin deposition. Age at presentation ranges from 14 to 77 years. There is a higher incidence in males (3:1).

T2-weighted MR images beautifully demonstrate thin lines of hypointense material along the surface of the brain. The findings are most striking along the brainstem and cerebellar vermis, as seen in this case. Low signal can also be seen along the cisternal portion of the cranial nerves and coating the spinal cord. Cerebellar atrophy is a common associated finding. Caution should be taken not to mistake the artifactual low-signal border at the brain/CSF interface seen on fast T2-weighted images for superficial siderosis. Intraventricular siderosis can occur following neonatal intraventricular hemorrhage and with intracranial vascular malformations and aneurysms.

Once superficial siderosis has been identified, it is important to evaluate the entire neuraxis to locate the inciting lesion. In the absence of an intracranial lesion, an ependymoma of the filum terminale should be searched for as the etiology of the recurrent hemorrhage. The only treatment is surgical resection of the bleeding source. In up to 50% of cases, the source of hemorrhage is never found.

SUGGESTED READINGS

Anderson NE, Sheffield S, Hope JK. Superficial siderosis of the CNS: a late complication of cerebellar tumors. *Neurology* 1999;52:163–169.

Fearnly JM, Stevens JM, Rudge P. Superficial siderosis of the CNS. *Brain* 1995;118:1051–1066.

Janss AG, Galetta SL, Freese A, et al. Superficial siderosis of the CNS: magnetic resonance imaging and pathologic correlation. Case report. *J Neurosurg* 1993;79:756–760.

Mamourian AC. MR of superficial siderosis. *AJNR* 1993;14:1445–1448.

Offenbacher H, Fazekas F, Schmidt R, et al. Superficial siderosis of the CNS: MRI findings and clinical significance. *Neuroradiology* 1996;38(Suppl):551–556.

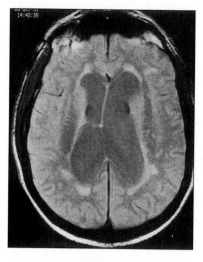

FIGURE 3.1A

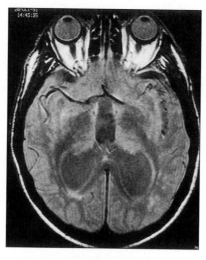

FIGURE 3.1B

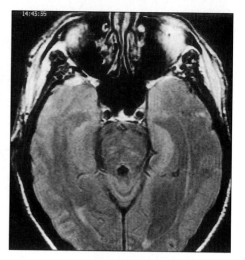

FIGURE 3.1C

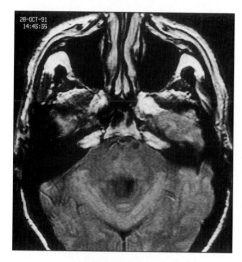

FIGURE 3.1D

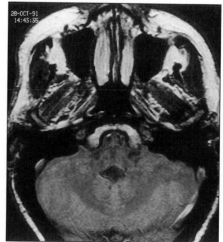

FIGURE 3.1E

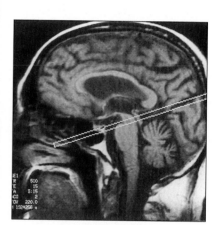

FIGURE 3.1F

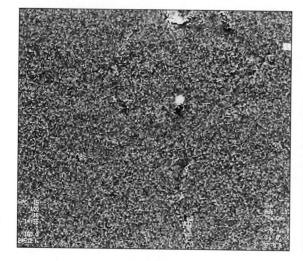

FIGURE 3.1G

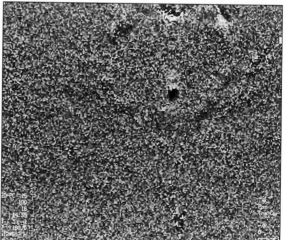

FIGURE 3.1H

CLINICAL HISTORY

A 78-year-old male with a history of ataxia, mild urinary incontinence, and short-term memory deficit.

FINDINGS

Proton-density-weighted MR images demonstrate enlargement of the ventricular system out of proportion to sulcal enlargement (Fig. 3.1A–E) with marked cerebrospinal fluid (CSF) flow void. CSF flow study (Fig. 3.1F–H) shows hyperdynamic CSF flow.

DIAGNOSIS

Normal pressure hydrocephalus (NPH).

DISCUSSION

Early clinical applications of MRI involving CSF motion were in the setting of hyperdynamic flow (e.g., communicating hydrocephalus), as well as complete obstruction (e.g., aqueductal stenosis with subsequent loss of the normal CSF flow void). More recently, it was shown that the extent of the aqueduct CSF flow void correlates well with favorable response to ventriculoperitoneal shunting for elderly patients with a form of communicating hydrocephalus known as *normal pressure hydrocephalus* (NPH) (Fig. 3.1A–E). In a related article, it was suggested that the gait disturbance of NPH results from the combination of tangential shearing forces and deep white matter ischemia (which affect the descending corticospinal white matter tracts abutting the lateral ventricles). When the CSF flow void noted on routine ungated MR images is pronounced, it suggests that symptomatic patients with NPH still have an intact blood supply to the brain (since systolic expansion of the cerebral hemispheres produces the CSF motion in the first place). When central atrophy develops, the blood supply to the brain is reduced, leading to decreased systolic expansion and subsequent reduction in the CSF flow.

Phase contrast techniques have been developed for quantitatively measuring CSF flow through the aqueduct. Using a 512 × 512 matrix over a 16-cm field of view, 0.32 mm pixels can be generated. A single-angled axial slice can be positioned perpendicular to the aqueduct and, using an encoding velocity (V_{enc}) of 200 mm/sec, CSF velocity can be measured (Fig. 3F–H). On phase contrast MR images systolic flow down appears white (Fig. 3.1G) and diastolic flow up appears black (Fig. 2.3H). By multiplying the velocity by the cross-sectional area of the aqueduct, the volumetric flow rate can be determined. Integrating over systole or diastole yields the volume of CSF flowing up and down over the cardiac cycle (i.e., the aqueductal CSF stroke volume). In a recent series, all NPH patients with a stroke volume greater than 42 μl responded to shunting compared with only 50% of those with CSF stroke volumes less than 42 μl.

Submitted by Sattam Lingawi, MB, ChB; Peter Brotchie, MBBS, PhD, FRCPC; William G. Bradley, MD, PhD, FACR (Senior Editor), Long Beach Memorial Medical Center, Long Beach, CA.

SUGGESTED READINGS

Bradley WG, Scalzo D, Queralt J, et al. Normal pressure hydrocephalus: evaluation with cerebrospinal fluid flow measurements at MR imaging. *Radiology* 1995;198:523–530.

Bradley WG, Whittemore AR, Kortman KE, et al. Marked CSF flow void: an indicator of successful shunting in patients with suspected normal pressure hydrocephalus. *Radiology* 1991;178:459–466.

Bradley WG, Whittemore AR, Watanabe AS, et al. Association of deep white matter infarction with chronic communicating hydrocephalus: implications regarding the possible origin of normal pressure hydrocephalus. *AJNR* 1991;12:31–39.

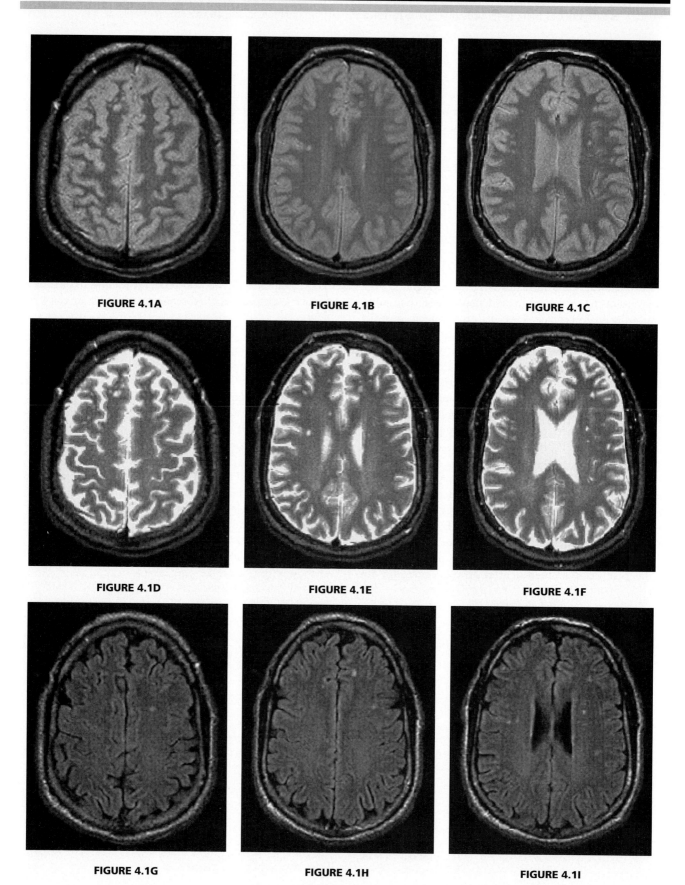

FIGURE 4.1A

FIGURE 4.1B

FIGURE 4.1C

FIGURE 4.1D

FIGURE 4.1E

FIGURE 4.1F

FIGURE 4.1G

FIGURE 4.1H

FIGURE 4.1I

CLINICAL HISTORY

A 37-year-old female with a clinical history of migraine headaches.

FINDINGS

Axial MR images demonstrate small, well-defined, hyperintense foci in the corona radiata and centrum semiovale of both cerebral hemispheres on proton density (Fig. 4.1A–C), T2-weighted (Fig. 4.1D–F), and fluid attenuated in version recovery (FLAIR) images (Fig. 4.1G–I).

DIAGNOSIS

Migraine.

DISCUSSION

Early periventricular abnormalities of any etiology may be difficult to detect on CT since they appear hypointense adjacent to the hypointense cerebrospinal fluid (CSF). By proper selection of TR and TE (repetition time and echo delay time, respectively) on MRI, the CSF can be made hypo- to isointense to brain, and periventricular white matter abnormalities are shown as hyperintensities. Thus MR is much more sensitive than CT in the detection of early noncalcified periventricular abnormalities. The differential diagnosis of these abnormalities depends heavily on the patient's age and clinical history.

Migraine is one cause of periventricular hyperintensities in young patients. These are believed to represent small, deep white matter infarcts due to an associated vasculitis. Other causes of vasculitis, particularly systemic lupus erythematosus, should also be included in the differential diagnosis.

The most likely cause of periventricular hyperintensities in young patients is multiple sclerosis (MS). MS lesions tend to be small, well defined, and ovoid; they often abut the lateral ventricles. They often involve the corpus callosum, brainstem, brachium pontis, and spinal cord. Acute disseminated encephalomyelitis (ADEM) is another entity that can result in a pattern similar to MS in this age group; however, unlike MS, it does not recur.

The most likely cause of periventricular hyperintensities in the elderly is ischemia. Larger lesions, particularly those at the gray–white matter junction, may be associated with cavitation, which produces CSF intensity on T1-weighted and FLAIR images. When cavitation is seen, deep white matter infarction is present (by definition). It is common to use the term *ischemic gliosis* to refer to the noncavitating diffuse periventricular abnormalities in these patients. In comparison with MS, ischemic lesions tend to be large and ill defined and are most commonly seen in the watershed distribution around the ventricles and the basal ganglia (supplied by the thalamoperforators and lenticulostriate arteries). This process is relatively ubiquitous, occurring in about 30% to 60% of patients more than 60 years of age. It is more commonly seen among smokers and diabetics and patients with hyperlipidemia.

Submitted by Peter Brotchie, MBBS, PhD; Sattam Lingawi, MB, ChB, FRCPC; William G. Bradley, MD, PhD, FACR (Senior Editor), Long Beach Memorial Medical Center, Long Beach, CA.

SUGGESTED READINGS

Bradley WG, et al. Use of ultra thin T1-weighted images to distinguish periventricular gliosis from deep white matter infarction. *Radiology* 1991;181:164.
Soges LJ, Cacayorin ED, Petro GR, et al. Migraine: evaluation of MR. *AJNR* 1988;9:425.

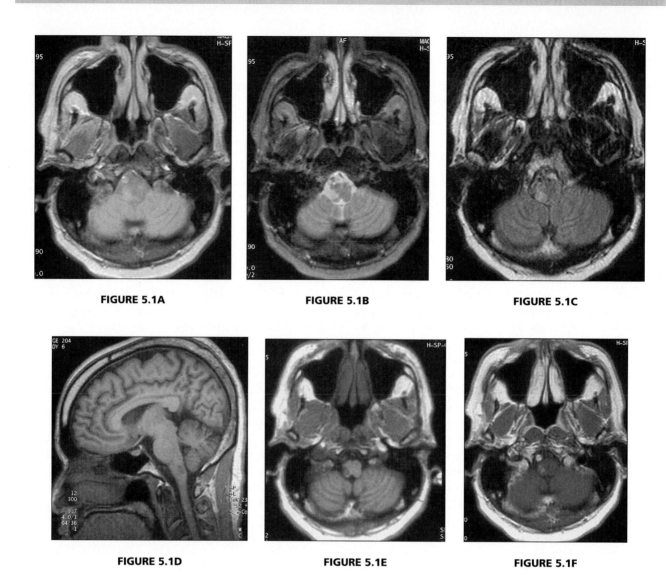

FIGURE 5.1A   **FIGURE 5.1B**   **FIGURE 5.1C**

FIGURE 5.1D   **FIGURE 5.1E**   **FIGURE 5.1F**

CLINICAL HISTORY

A 51-year-old male with recent onset of right facial and left body numbness, and ptosis, miosis, and anhydrosis on the right.

FINDINGS

High signal is noted on the axial proton-density and T2-weighted (Fig. 5.1A,B) and FLAIR (Fig. 5.1C) images through the right lateral aspect of the medulla. High signal within the right vertebral artery on the unenhanced sagittal T1-weighted image (Fig. 5.1D) and enhancement (Fig. 5E,F) following administration of contrast suggest very slow flow. Enhancement is also noted in the lesion.

DIAGNOSIS

Subacute lateral medullary infarct.

DISCUSSION

The normal appearance of large arteries on spin-echo images is low signal (i.e., the classic "flow void"). An exception to this statement occurs when vessels are caught in cross section upon first entering an imaging volume. High signal on the entry slices represents flow-related enhancement due to inflow of unsaturated spins. (This is the phenomenon responsible for time-of-flight MR angiography.) Although high signal may occasionally be seen for through-plane flow, it is rarely seen in arteries flowing within the plane (e.g., the orientation of the right vertebral artery on the sagittal view). This finding is worrisome for abnormally slow flow or thrombosis. The subsequent enhancement with gadolinium supports a diagnosis of very slow flow rather than complete thrombosis. Since the lateral aspect of the medulla is fed by branches of the posterior inferior cerebellar artery, which arises from the vertebral artery, the process of clotting and unclotting beyond a stenosis is the likely cause of this medullary infarct.

Wallenberg's syndrome is a composite of symptoms arising from involvement of the white matter tracts and nuclei in the lateral aspect of the medulla. The right-sided facial numbness results from involvement of the trigeminal spinal tract, which carries pain and temperature sensation from the ipsilateral face. The numbness on the left side of the body is due to involvement of the spinothalamic tracts, which also carry pain and temperature sensation. These tracts cross within two levels of entering the spine, explaining the contralateral symptoms. The ipsilateral Horner's syndrome (ptosis, miosis, and anhydrosis) is due to involvement of the sympathetic fibers descending from the brain that will eventually exit the spinal canal in the upper cervical region to ascend back into the brain along the carotid arteries. With larger medullary infarcts, there may be contralateral hemiparesis (due to involvement of the corticospinal tract) and there may be involvement of the nucleus ambiguous as well, leading to hoarseness (due to paralysis of the ipsilateral vocal cord) and difficulty swallowing (due to involvement of the superior constrictor muscles of the pharynx).

Submitted by William G. Bradley, MD, PhD, FACR (Senior Editor), Long Beach Memorial Medical Center, Long Beach, CA.

SUGGESTED READING

Bradley WG. Brainstem: normal anatomy and pathology. In: Stark DD, Bradley WG, eds. *Magnetic resonance imaging,* 3rd ed. St. Louis: Mosby, 1999:1187–1208.

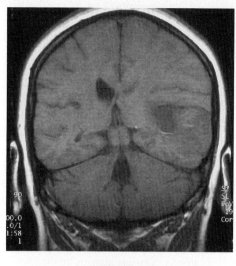

FIGURE 6.1A

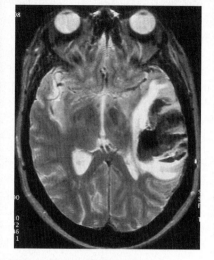

FIGURE 6.1B

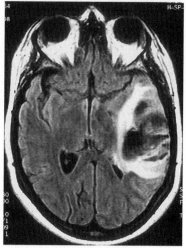

FIGURE 6.1C

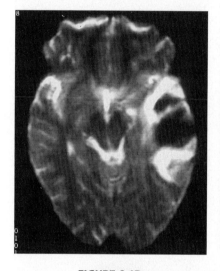

FIGURE 6.1D

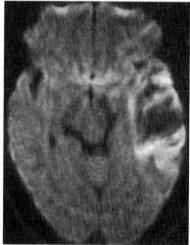

FIGURE 6.1E

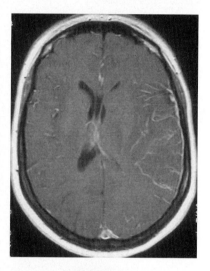

FIGURE 6.1F

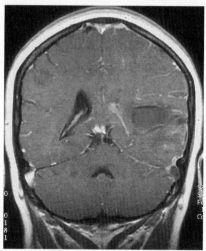
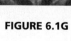

FIGURE 6.1G

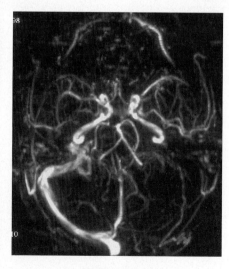

FIGURE 6.1H

CLINICAL HISTORY

A 33-year-old female presenting initially with severe headache and then right facial palsy and right hemiparesis.

FINDINGS

There is a large lesion in the left temporal lobe. It is surrounded by vasogenic edema, which is dark on the T1-weighted image (Fig. 6.1A) and quite conspicuous and bright on the T2-weighted and FLAIR images (Fig. 6.1B,C). The lesion itself is isointense to brain on the T1-weighted image and quite dark on the T2-weighted and FLAIR images. This low signal intensity is also noted on the ($b = 0$) image (Fig. 6.1D) of the echo planar imaging (EPI) diffusion study that persists on the ($b = 1,000$) diffusion image (Fig. 6.1E). Following administration of gadolinium, there is stasis over the left temporal lobe (Fig. 6.1F). While the right transverse sinus opacifies normally, there is no opacification of the left transverse sinus (Fig. 6.1G). On phase contrast MRA, there is no flow in the left transverse sinus (Fig. 6.1H).

DIAGNOSIS

Venous infarction (dural sinus thrombosis with secondary parenchymal hemorrhage).

DISCUSSION

The appearance of this hemorrhage (isointense to brain on a T1-weighted image and dark on the T2-weighted and FLAIR images) is consistent with hemorrhage 24 to 72 hours old. Acute hemorrhage consists of paramagnetic intracellular deoxyhemoglobin.

Venous infarction occurs as a result of thrombosis of a dural sinus with backup of venous blood into the capillary system, leading to venous enhancement and low-pressure parenchymal hemorrhage. In this case, the vein of Labbé (not shown), which normally drains this portion of the temporal lobe, cannot drain into the thrombosed left transverse sinus leading to temporal lobe hemorrhage. Since these are low-pressure bleeds, they tend to do better than high-pressure arterial bleeds (e.g., from ruptured aneurysms).

The predominantly low signal on the diffusion image reflects "negative T2 shinethrough". A diffusion image in general starts with the T2-weighted baseline EPI image ($b = 0$) and then superimposes diffusion effects ($b = 1,000$). (The b value is a measure of the sensitivity to diffusion.) When the $b = 0$ image has a particularly low-intensity (or high-intensity) area, as in this case, it can also show up dark (or bright) on the diffusion image ($b = 1,000$). This is T2 shinethrough (negative and positive, respectively). The rim of high signal intensity surrounding the low-intensity hematoma may represent ischemic changes at the interface between the hematoma and the normal brain, or it may represent a thin rim of extracellular methemoglobin (which is also bright on diffusion imaging).

Phase contrast MRA is recommended in cases of suspected dural sinus thrombosis instead of the usual time-of-flight MRA because bright methemoglobin can simulate flow in the latter.

Submitted by William G. Bradley, MD, PhD, FACR (Senior Editor), Long Beach Memorial Medical Center, Long Beach, CA.

SUGGESTED READINGS

Jensen MC, Brant-Zawadzki MN, Jacobs BC. Ischemia. In: Stark DD, Bradley WG, eds. *Magnetic resonance imaging*, 3rd ed. St. Louis: Mosby, 1999:1255–1276.

Masaryk TJ, Perl J, Dagirmanjian, et al. Magnetic resonance angiography: neuroradiological applications. In: Stark DD, Bradley WG, eds. *Magnetic resonance imaging*, 3rd ed. St. Louis: Mosby, 1999:1277–1316.

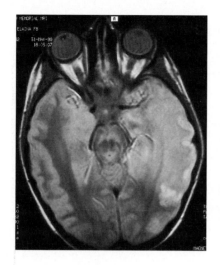

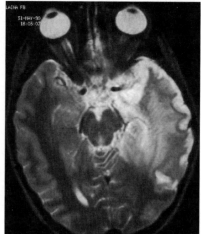

FIGURE 7.1A   **FIGURE 7.1B**

CLINICAL HISTORY

A previously healthy 8-year-old female who became comatose over several hours.

FINDINGS

Marked hyperintensity is noted on proton-density and T2-weighted images in the left temporal lobe (Fig. 7.1A,B).

DIAGNOSIS

Herpes encephalitis.

DISCUSSION

It is important to make the diagnosis of herpes encephalitis quickly, as it is treatable. Involvement of the temporal lobes is classic. Like other viral infections, herpes causes a meningoencephalitis. Thus the hyperintensity on MR scans tends to start peripherally in the meninges and cortex, and then progresses centrally. Note the involvement of the right temporal lobe, which is limited to the parahippocampal cortex, while the left temporal lobe disease has progressed into the white matter. This centripetal pattern helps to distinguish herpes encephalitis from acute disseminated encephalomyelitis (ADEM), a postviral leukoencephalopathy that may present with similar findings. Unlike herpes, ADEM affects the white matter first and then progresses centrifugally. The treatment for ADEM is also entirely different from that for herpes (i.e., steroids and plasmapheresis versus acyclovir). Thus MR should be used for the evaluation of these patients.

Submitted by William G. Bradley, MD, PhD, FACR (Senior Editor), Long Beach Memorial Medical Center, Long Beach, CA.

SUGGESTED READING

Sze GK. Infection and inflammation. In: Stark DD, Bradley WG, eds. *Magnetic resonance imaging*, 3rd ed. St. Louis: Mosby, 1999:1363–1378.

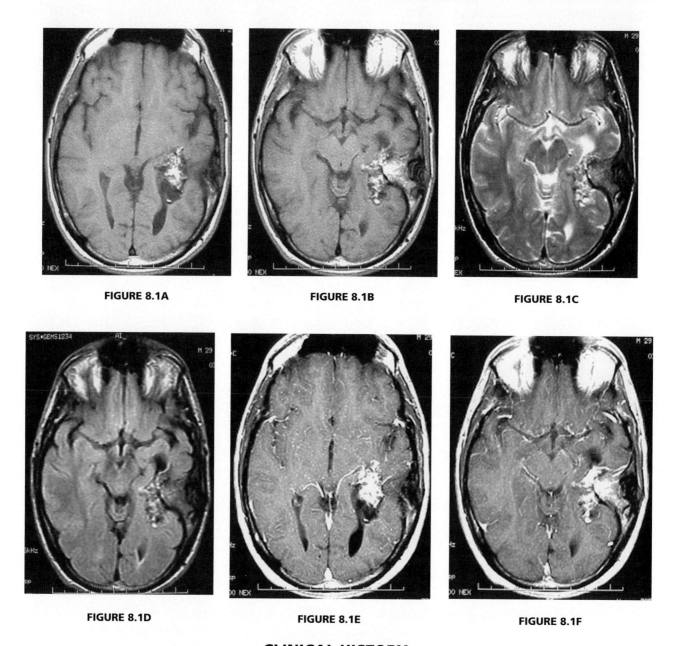

FIGURE 8.1A

FIGURE 8.1B

FIGURE 8.1C

FIGURE 8.1D

FIGURE 8.1E

FIGURE 8.1F

CLINICAL HISTORY

A 29-year-old male with history of headache.

FINDINGS

Axial noncontrast T1-weighted images (Fig. 8.1A,B) demonstrate large, lobulated mass extending from the left petrous apex into the left middle and posterior cranial fossa. There is mass effect upon the left lateral ventricle with entrapment of the temporal horn as well as compression of the left posterolateral aspect of the midbrain. The mass is hyperintense on the T1-weighted acquisition, similar in signal to the marrow within the adjacent petrous apex.

On T2-weighted and FLAIR acquisition (Fig. 8.1C,D), the mass is heterogeneous in signal. There is no abnormal signal within the adjacent brain parenchyma. There is no significant enhancement on postcontrast T1-weighted images (Fig. 8.1E,F).

DIAGNOSIS

Osteochondroma arising from the left petrous apex.

DISCUSSION

Osteochondroma is the most common benign bone tumor. It results from displaced growth plate cartilage that grows as an excrescence, usually from the metaphysis of long bones. There is usually continuity of the periosteum, cortices, and marrow extending into the exostosis from host bone. A cartilaginous cap covers the exostosis, which is the source of growth. Osteochondromas may extend from the host bone on a stalk (pedunculated lesion) or in a broad-based, sessile fashion. Most osteochondromas are found in the extremities. The most frequent site is around the knee.

Intracranial osteochondromas are very rare. They typically arise from bones that are derived from cartilage; therefore intracranial lesions have a predilection for the skull base. There is heterogeneous signal on T1- and T2-weighted images. A typical "honeycomb" appearance is attributed to a mixture of soft tissue and calcification. A heterogeneous calcified mass is seen on CT. There is usually no enhancement.

Surgical resection is the treatment of choice and the overall prognosis is good. Malignant transformation is rare isolitary lesions. In hereditary multiple exostosis, there is a 15% incidence of malignant degeneration.

SUGGESTED READINGS

Beck DW, Dyste GN. Intracranial osteochondroma: MR and CT appearance. *AJNR* 1989;10:S7–S8.
Berkmen YM, Blatt ES. Cranial and intracranial cartilaginous tumours. *Clin Radiol* 1968;19:327–333.

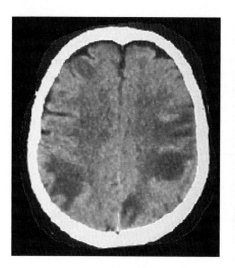

FIGURE 9.1A

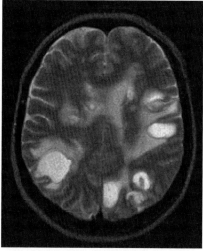

FIGURE 9.1B

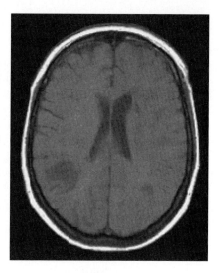

FIGURE 9.1C

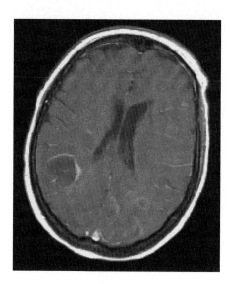

FIGURE 9.1D

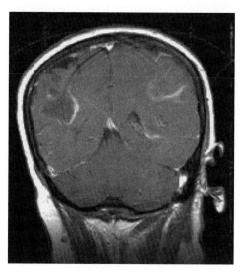

FIGURE 9.1E

CLINICAL HISTORY

A 35-year-old female with generalized fatigue and history of previous optic neuritis.

FINDINGS

Unenhanced CT image demonstrates widespread areas of hypodensity within the deep cerebral white matter with associated vasogenic edema (Fig. 9.1A). T2-weighted MR image shows a "fried egg" appearance of white matter lesions with surrounding vasogenic edema (Fig. 9.1B). The lesions are hypointense on T1-weighted images (Fig. 9.1C) with partial ring enhancement (Fig. 9.1D,E).

DIAGNOSIS

Tumefactive multiple sclerosis.

DISCUSSION

Multiple sclerosis (MS) is a disease of young people (i.e., the same population generally affected by primary gliomas). Both can present as an acute or insidious process. Acute tumefactive MS is bright on T2-weighted images, enhances with gadolinium, and exerts mass effect on the surrounding structures. Note that the enhancement is most marked on the medial aspect of the lesions, reflecting the vascular supply, another feature typical of MS plaques. The fried egg appearance is virtually diagnostic of acute tumefactive multiple sclerosis. When it occurs as an isolated process, however, it may be impossible to distinguish MS from a primary neoplasm. When found in combination with additional white matter lesions, the diagnosis of multiple sclerosis can be suggested. This is particularly true when such lesions have the typical ovoid configuration with the long axis perpendicular to the walls of the lateral ventricles. Clinically, both acute tumefactive MS and tumors can present insidiously; however, a history of previous transient neurologic deficits is suggestive of MS. When the diagnosis is uncertain it is useful to delay biopsy for a period of 6 to 12 weeks. During this time, acute tumefactive MS should begin to decrease in size or degree of enhancement while tumors will stay the same or increase.

Submitted by Sattam Lingawi, MB, ChB; Peter Brotchie, MBBS, PhD, FRCPC; William G. Bradley, MD, PhD, FACR (Senior Editor), Long Beach Memorial Medical Center, Long Beach, CA.

SUGGESTED READINGS

Dagher AP, Smirniotopoulos J. Tumefactive demyelinating diseases. *Neuroradiology* 1996;38:560–565.
Horowitz AL, Kaplan RD, Grewe G, et al. The ovoid lesion: a new MR observation in patients with multiple sclerosis. *Am J Neuroradiol* 1989;10:303.

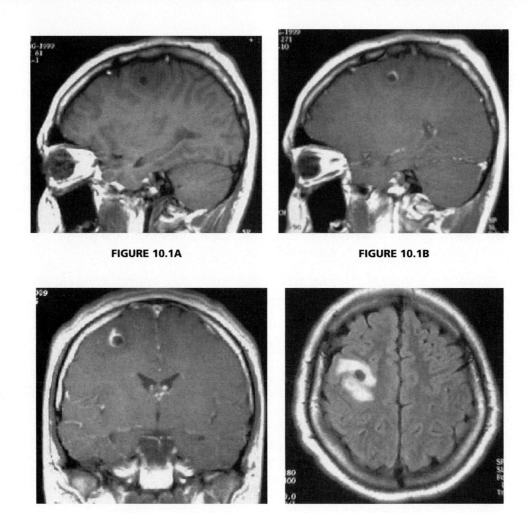

FIGURE 10.1A   FIGURE 10.1B

FIGURE 10.1C   FIGURE 10.1D

CLINICAL HISTORY

A 27-year-old male from Mexico with headache and visual disturbance.

FINDINGS

T1-weighted and FLAIR images demonstrate a small, cystic lesion with surrounding edema (Fig. 10.1A,D). Peripheral enhancement is evident on the postcontrast T1-weighted images (Fig. 10.1B,C).

DIAGNOSIS

Cysticercosis.

DISCUSSION

Cysticercosis is a parasitic infestation caused by the pork tapeworm (*Tenia solium*). It gains access to the human body in the form of a tapeworm egg that is ingested in partially cooked food or drinks. Gastric acid dissolves the eggshell, and the embryo (oncosphere) is released into the intestine. It penetrates the intestinal wall and disseminates into the human body (definitive host), preferentially lodging in the brain (80%), eyes, and muscles. There the embryos develop into larvae in 8 to 12 weeks.

Within the brain the cysticerci may be leptomeningeal, parenchymal, or intraventricular. As they develop they form a cystic mass with (*Cysticercus cellulosae*) or without (*Cysticercus racemosus*) a scolex. The latter form is usually present in the subarachnoid space, particularly the basal cisterns. Symptoms vary according to the location of the lesions. The subarachnoid involvement often results in intense meningeal reaction, causing cranial neuropathy and vasculopathy.

The lesions are generally asymptomatic while the parasite is alive. However, as it starts to die, it incites an intense local-tissue reaction with associated neurologic sequelae. With proper medical therapy these lesions eventually shrink and calcify.

Submitted by Peter Brotchie, MBBS, PhD; Sattam Lingawi, MB, ChB, FRCPC; William G. Bradley, MD, PhD, FACR (Senior Editor), Long Beach Memorial Medical Center, Long Beach, CA.

SUGGESTED READINGS

Bia FJ, Barry M. Parasitic infections of the central nervous system. *Neurol Clin* 1986;4:171.

Suss RA, Maravilla KR, Thompson J. MR imaging of intracranial cysticercosis: comparison with CT and anatomopathologic features. *Am J Neuroradiol* 1986;7:235.

Zee CS, Segall HD, Apuzzo MLJ, et al. Intraventricular cysticercal cysts: further neuroradiologic observations and neurosurgical implications. *Am J Neuroradiol* 1984;5:727.

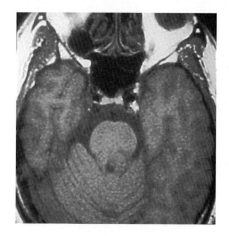

FIGURE 11.1A

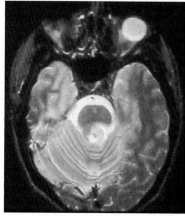

FIGURE 11.1B

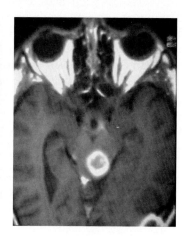

FIGURE 11.1C

CLINICAL HISTORY

A 35-year-old male presents with right-sided weakness and visual disturbance.

FINDINGS

Axial T1- and T2-weighted images (Fig. 11.1A,B) demonstrate a rounded lesion with perifocal edema involving the dorsal and left lateral aspect of the pons in the region of the superior cerebellar peduncle. The lesion is isointense to brain parenchyma on T1-weighted acquisition and slightly hyperintense on T2-weighted images. Following intravenous contrast (Fig. 11.1C), there is intense, nodular, ring enhancement. (Figure 11.1A courtesy of Tufail Patankar, MD, Manchester, England.)

DIAGNOSIS

Tuberculoma.

DISCUSSION

In recent years, the incidence of tuberculosis (TB) is rising, particularly among immigrants, the homeless, IV drug abusers, those who are infected by HIV, and institutionalized patients. *Mycobacterium tuberculosis* is the responsible organism in the vast majority of cases. *Mycobacterium avium-intracellulare* complex rarely involves the central nervous system (CNS). Most adult CNS TB is a postprimary infection, whereas in children, it is usually part of a primary infection. CNS TB occurs in 2% to 5% of all patients with TB and in 10% of those with AIDS-related TB infection. In postprimary infection, it is postulated that the organism is transported to the meninges and/or brain parenchyma hematogenously from a primary pulmonary tuberculous infection. Coexistent pulmonary TB is seen in 25% to 83% of cases of CNS TB.

Various manifestations of CNS TB include TB meningitis, parenchymal abscess, focal cerebritis, and tuberculoma (demonstrated in this case). Tuberculoma is the most common manifestation of CNS parenchymal TB infection. Histologically, tuberculomas are granulomas with central caseous necrosis. They most frequently occur in the cerebral hemispheres (at the corticomedullary junction and in the periventricular region) and basal ganglia in adults and in the cerebellum in children. The ventricles and brainstem are less commonly involved. The subarachnoid, subdural, and epidural space can also be affected. Tuberculomas are usually solitary but can be multiple in 10% to 35% of cases. A miliary pattern of disease is uncommon, except in the pediatric population. Parenchymal disease can occur with or without concomitant meningeal disease.

In the acute stage, tuberculomas are iso- to slightly hyperdense ill-defined masses on noncontrast CT with irregular ring or nodular enhancement following contrast. Mature tuberculomas are well-defined round or oval ring-enhancing lesions. One-third of patients will demonstrate "target" lesions, which appear as peripherally enhancing lesions with central focus of calcification or enhancement. This finding is suggestive of the tuberculoma but not specific for the disease. On MRI, tuberculomas are iso- to hypointense on T1-weighted images. They occasionally feature a rim of high signal. Lesions are typically hypointense on T2-weighted images, although the greater the degree of central necrosis, the more hyperintense the lesion. There is intense nodular or ringlike enhancement following contrast. Perilesional mass effect and edema are usually present, typically more prominent in the early stages of granuloma formation. Healed lesions often calcify and are more easily identified on CT than MRI.

Tuberculous abscess is a rare complication of CNS TB. The abscesses are usually larger than tuberculomas and have a more accelerated clinical course. The appearance is similar to pyogenic abscess but is more often multiloculated.

The differential diagnosis for a solitary tuberculoma includes abscess, astrocytoma, or metastasis. A cysticercus lesion can have similar imaging features but is typically smaller than tuberculoma.

SUGGESTED READINGS

Chang K-H, Han M-H, Roh J-K, et al. Gd-DTPA enhanced MR imaging in intracranial tuberculosis. *Neuroradiology* 1991;238:340–344.

Gupta RK, Jena A, Sharma DK, et al. MR imaging of intracranial tuberculomas. *JCAT* 1988;12:280–285.

Hansman Whiteman ML, Bowen BC, Donovan Post MJ, et al. Intracranial infection. In: Atlas SW, ed. *Magnetic resonance imaging of the brain and spine*, 2nd ed. Philadelphia: Lippincott-Raven, 1996:738–742.

Jinkins JR. Computed tomography of intracranial tuberculosis. *Neuroradiology* 1991;33:126–135.

Kloumehr F, Dadsetan MR, Rooholamini SA, et al. Central nervous system tuberculosis: MRI. *Neuroradiology* 1994;36:93–96.

Sheller JR, Des Prez RM. CNS tuberculosis. *Neurol Clin* 1986;4:143–158.

Tyson G, Newman P, Strachen WE. Tuberculous brain abscess. *Surg Neurol* 1978;10:323–325.

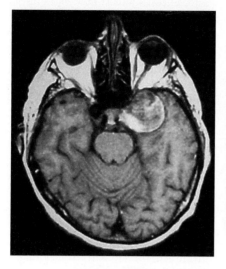

FIGURE 12.1A

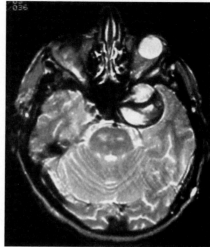

FIGURE 12.1B

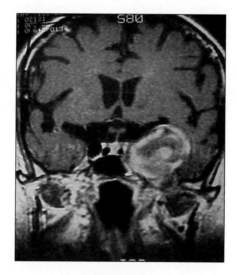

FIGURE 12.1C

CLINICAL HISTORY

A 73-year-old female with history of left sixth nerve palsy.

FINDINGS

Axial noncontrast T1-weighted acquisition (Fig. 12.1A) demonstrates a large, well-defined, rounded extraaxial mass extending from the left cavernous sinus into the middle cranial fossa. There is heterogeneous, predominantly hyperintense signal within this lesion. Axial T2-weighted acquisition (Fig. 12.1B) shows heterogeneous signal within this mass. There is a well-defined hypointense rim. There is no definite enhancement of this mass on postcontrast coronal T1-weighted acquisition (Fig. 12.1C). The mass appears to arise from the cavernous left internal carotid artery, which is not identified as a separate structure. Note fusiform dilation of the cavernous right internal carotid artery. Note also phase-shift artifact in the phase-encoded direction (left to right), confirming that this is a vascular lesion. Incidental note is made of punctate focus of high signal within the pons on axial T2-weighted acquisition suggestive of ischemic change. (Courtesy of William Greenlee, MD, Rush-Presbyterian-St. Luke's Medical Center, Chicago, Illinois.)

DIAGNOSIS

Giant aneurysm of the cavernous left internal carotid artery.

DISCUSSION

Cerebral aneurysms are found in up to 14% of the population. There are two major forms of aneurysm, saccular and fusiform. Saccular aneurysms are true aneurysms. They are focal dilatations of the vascular lumen due to weakness of all three-vessel wall layers. The wall of the aneurysm is composed of intima and adventitia; the media is typically thinned or absent. In saccular aneurysms the dome of the lesion is wider than the neck. Fusiform aneurysms are an exaggerated, irregular ectasia of the involved vessel. The common proposed etiologies for intracranial aneurysm include hemodynamically induced degenerative vascular injury, atherosclerosis (typically fusiform aneurysms), underlying vasculopathy (i.e., fibromuscular dysplasia, Marfan's syndrome), or high-flow states (i.e., arteriovenous malformations). Less common causes are trauma, infection, drug abuse, and neoplasm.

Giant aneurysms by definition are those aneurysms that are greater than 2.5 cm in diameter; invariably, they are of the saccular type. They are most commonly found in middle-aged women. Giant aneurysms typically present as mass lesions with symptoms related to perilesional mass effect, as opposed to smaller aneurysms, which typically present with subarachnoid hemorrhage. Subarachnoid hemorrhage does, however, occur. The most frequent presenting complaint is cranial neuropathy. Seizures, ischemia, and endocrinologic disturbances can be seen.

Most giant aneurysms are located along the extradural internal carotid artery (ICA), within the cavernous ICA or middle cerebral artery. The anterior cerebral artery and vertebrobasilar arteries are the next most common locations.

Most giant aneurysms are partially thrombosed. Complete thrombotic occlusion can also occur. The characteristic MRI feature of a giant aneurysm is a well-defined mass lesion with laminated thrombus consisting of layers of mixed signal intensities (reflecting various stages of blood degradation). There is flow void within the patent portion of the lumen and often high signal around the patent lumen reflecting slow-flowing blood and/or methemoglobin. Hemorrhage and edema are rarely seen in the surrounding brain parenchyma. Enhancement is variable; the patent residual lumen will typically enhance. Subarachnoid hemorrhage, if present, is difficult to identify on MRI, although FLAIR images can occasionally make the diagnosis. (See Vol. 1, Case 18.)

Flowing blood (signal void) within a complex signal mass is pathognomonic for aneurysm. Ghost image pulsation artifact (in the phase-encoding direction) is an important observation defining these lesions. A high-density mass is seen on noncontrast CT. Calcification is common.

MRA can be useful in the diagnosis; however, giant aneurysms can be missed because of saturation of slow intraluminal flow and/or thrombosis, particularly on three-dimensional time-of-flight (TOF) images. Another pitfall of MRA is that high-signal thrombus can be misinterpreted as flowing blood. MRA should not be interpreted without an accompanying MRI in the evaluation of giant aneurysm. MRI has been reported to be the best screening tool for partially or completely thrombosed aneurysms. The aneurysm size, location, and associated mass effect can be determined. Catheter angiography is limiting in that only the patent portion of the aneurysm can be seen.

SUGGESTED READINGS

Biondi A, Scialta G, Scotti G. Intracranial aneurysms: MR imaging. *Neuroradiology* 1988;30:214–218.

De Jesus O, Ritkinson N. MR angiography of giant aneurysms: pitfalls and surgical implications. *P R Health Sci J* 1997;16:131–135.

Lang EW, Steffens JC, Link J, et al. The utility of contrast enhancement MR angiography for posterior fossa giant cerebral aneurysm management. *Neurol Res* 1998;20:705–708.

Matsumura K, Saito A, Nakasu Y, et al. MR imaging of large and giant intracranial aneurysms. *Neurol Med Chir (Tokyo)* 1990;30:382–388.

Vorkapic P, Czech T, Pendl G, et al. Clinico-radiological spectrum of giant intracranial aneurysms. *Neurosurg Rev* 1991;14:271–274.

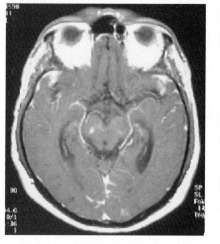

FIGURE 13.1A

FIGURE 13.1B

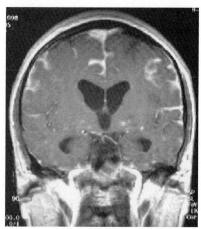
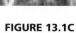

FIGURE 13.1C

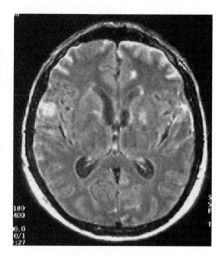

FIGURE 13.1D

CLINICAL HISTORY

A 72-year-old female with blood-tinged vaginal discharge for 3 months now presents with seizures.

FINDINGS

Postcontrast T1-weighted (Fig. 13.1A–C) and FLAIR (Fig. 13.1D) images demonstrate thickened enhancing regions along the brain surface, extending into the sulci and interhemispheric fissure.

DIAGNOSIS

Leptomeningeal metastases.

DISCUSSION

Leptomeningeal metastases (i.e., to the pia and arachnoid) are common and may be the only finding in 18% of intracranial metastases. Leptomeningeal metastases occur via hematogenous spread through meningeal and choroidal vessels. From there metastasis may extend along the Virchow-Robin spaces and produce an appearance simulating intraparenchymal disease.

Adult tumors that commonly involve the leptomeninges are bronchogenic carcinoma, breast carcinoma, lymphoma, and astrocytomas. A similar metastatic pattern is usually seen in childhood with leukemia, ependymoma, primitive neuroectodermal tumor (PNET), and neuroblastoma. Contrast-enhanced T1-weighted MR images have become an important adjunct to cerebrospinal fluid (CSF) analysis with greater than 70% sensitivity for detection of metastatic spread. This sensitivity is even higher with the application of MRI techniques such as higher-dose gadolinium, enhanced FLAIR, and enhanced T1-weighted images with magnetization transfer.

The dura (i.e., the pachymeninges) normally shows minimal enhancement with a thin (under 1 mm), linear, smooth, interrupted appearance that does not extend into the sulci. Leptomeningeal metastases often cause enhancement of long segments of thickened meninges or may appear as enhancing nodules with extension into the sulci. Tumor may also coat the leptomeninges and enhance in a smooth but diffuse pattern (called *zücherguss,* or sugar coating) that may not be easily differentiated from other causes such as inflammatory or infectious processes.

Submitted by Sattam Lingawi, MB, ChB; Peter Brotchie, MBBS, PhD, FRCPC; William G. Bradley, MD, PhD, FACR (Senior Editor), Long Beach Memorial Medical Center, Long Beach, CA.

SUGGESTED READINGS

Delatter JY, Krol G, Thalr HT, et al. Distribution of brain metastasis. *Arch Neurol* 1988;45:741.
Laws ERJ, Thapar K. Brain tumors. *Cancer* 1993;43:262.

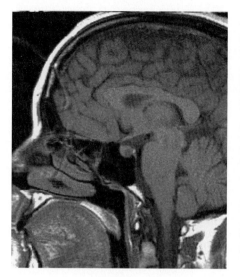

FIGURE 14.1A

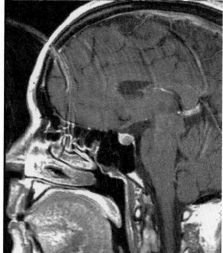

FIGURE 14.1B

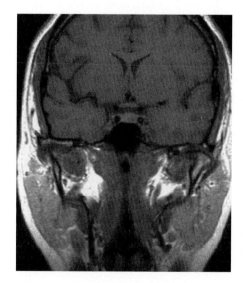

FIGURE 14.1C

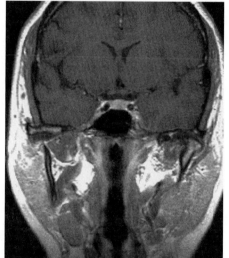

FIGURE 14.1D

CLINICAL HISTORY

A 35-year-old female with Cushing's disease.

FINDINGS

A 9-mm hypointense rounded lesion is evident in the pituitary gland on sagittal and coronal T1-weighted images (Fig. 14.1A,C). The lesion enhances poorly relative to the rest of the pituitary gland (Fig. 14.1B,D).

DIAGNOSIS

Pituitary microadenoma.

DISCUSSION

Pituitary microadenomas are benign tumors of the anterior lobe of the pituitary gland (adenohypophysis) that measure less than 10 mm in size. These tumors are usually hormonally active. Depending on the cell type, they may produce prolactin, adrenocorticotrophic hormone (ACTH), or growth hormone leading to amenorrhea/galactorrhea, Cushing's disease, or acromegaly/gigantism, respectively.

MRI is preferable to CT for pituitary imaging due to its superior soft-tissue contrast and absence of beam-hardening artifact. Typically, 3-mm T1-weighted conventional spin-echo images are acquired in the coronal and sagittal planes. Dynamic pituitary imaging (i.e., a precontrast T1-weighted fast spin echo followed by early and late postcontrast scanning) may be of use. Such a protocol takes advantage of the natural tumor pattern of enhancement, which lags behind the normal pituitary gland in both contrast uptake and release. This results in the visualization of the microadenoma as a hypointense intrapituitary mass in the early scan that turns hyperintense (relative to the pituitary gland) on the delayed scan.

The differential diagnosis in the setting of hormonal activity is virtually nonexistent. However, if the patient is asymptomatic, a pars intermedia cyst, Rathke's cleft cyst, or pituitary metastasis may need to be considered.

Submitted by Peter Brotchie, MBBS, PhD; Sattam Lingawi, MB, ChB, FRCPC; William G. Bradley, MD, PhD, FACR (Senior Editor), Long Beach Memorial Medical Center, Long Beach, CA.

SUGGESTED READINGS

Davis PC, Gokhale KA, Joseph GJ, et al. Pituitary adenoma: correlation of half-dose gadolinium-enhanced MR imaging with surgical findings in 26 patients. *Radiology* 1991;180:779.

Finelli DA, Kaufman B. Varied microcirculation of pituitary adenomas at rapid, dynamic, contrast-enhanced MR imaging. *Radiology* 1993;189:205.

Kucharczyk W, Davis DO, Kelly WM, et al. Pituitary adenomas: high-resolution MR imaging at 1.5 T. *Radiology* 1986;161:761.

Molitch ME, Russell EJ. The pituitary "incidentaloma." *Ann Intern Med* 1990;112:925.

Newton DR, Dillon WP, Norman D, et al. Gd-DTPA-enhanced MR imaging of pituitary adenomas. *AJNR* 1988;10:949.

Yuh WTC, et al. Sequential MR enhancement pattern in normal pituitary gland and in pituitary adenoma. *AJNR* 1994;15:101.

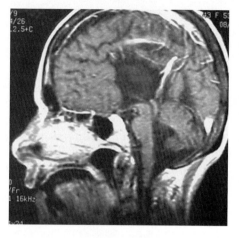

FIGURE 15.1A **FIGURE 15.1B**

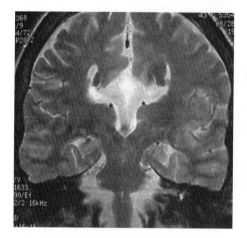

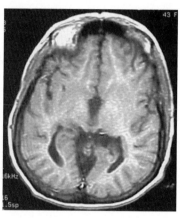
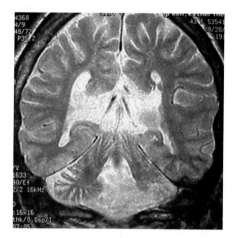

FIGURE 15.1C **FIGURE 15.1D** **FIGURE 15.1E**

CLINICAL HISTORY

A 43-year-old female with seizures.

FINDINGS

Midline sagittal postcontrast T1-weighted acquisition (Fig. 15.1A) shows absence of the corpus callosum. Note absence of the cingulate gyrus. The cortical sulci extend directly to the ventricular surface. Axial T1-weighted image (Fig. 15.1B) demonstrates the parallel configuration of the lateral ventricles as well as a high-riding third ventricle. Coronal T2-weighted images (Fig. 15.1C) demonstrate white matter tracts coursing along the medial aspect of the lateral ventricles, known as Bundles of Probst. Note the classic "steer head" sign used to describe the configuration of ventricles on the coronal acquisition. Axial T1- and coronal T2-weighted images through the atria of the lateral ventricles (Fig. 15.1D,E) show multiple subependymal nodules, which are isointense with cortical gray matter consistent with nodular heterotopia.

DIAGNOSIS

Agenesis of corpus callosum with nodular heterotopia.

DISCUSSION

The corpus callosum is composed of four segments: the rostrum, genu, body, and splenium. The corpus callosum forms from anterior to posterior with the exception of the rostrum (the anterior and inferior portion of the corpus callosum, which connects the genu and the lamina terminalis), which forms last. Callosal anomalies range from agenesis (seen in this case) to partial absence (or hypogenesis). When only partially absent, the splenium and rostrum of the corpus callosum are almost always missing. The genu and body are usually present to various degrees. The exception to the rule is in the setting of holoprosencephaly, where the splenium may be present in the absence of the genu and/or body. In holoprosencephaly, the corpus callosum is "dysgenetic" or malformed, as opposed to the more common incompletely formed or absent corpus callosum.

The corpus callosum normally forms during the period between 8 and 20 weeks of gestation. Most of the cerebrum and cerebellum is forming at the same time; therefore anomalies of the corpus callosum are often associated with other brain anomalies. Commonly associated anomalies include Dandy-Walker malformation, Chiari II malformation, gray matter heterotopias (as seen in this case), encephaloceles, holoprosencephaly, azygous anterior cerebral artery, midline facial anomalies, and "callosal" or pericallosal lipoma. (See Vol. 2, Case 61.) There is a strong association with Aicardi syndrome (females with agenesis of the corpus callosum, ocular abnormalities, and infantile spasms).

Isolated agenesis of the corpus callosum is usually asymptomatic and is found incidentally when imaging the brain for other reasons. When patients with callosal anomalies are symptomatic, it is typically the associated anomalies that are the cause of the symptoms. Common presenting symptoms include seizures, mental retardation, macrocephaly, and hypothalamic dysfunction.

The multiplanar capability of MRI is advantageous in imaging callosal anomalies. Although they can be detected in the axial plane, the sagittal and coronal planes are better for demonstrating the associated anatomic deformities.

In agenesis of the corpus callosum, the lateral ventricles are widely separated and parallel to each other as opposed to their normal convergent configuration. The lateral ventricles manifest a classic contour abnormality characterized by small, pointed frontal horns with asymmetrically enlarged occipital horns (colpocephaly). On coronal images, prominent bands of white matter invaginate the medial border of the lateral ventricles (most pronounced in the frontal horns). These white matter tracts are known as *Probst's bundles* and are longitudinally oriented axons that would have normally crossed into the contralateral hemisphere via the corpus callosum but that, in its absence, turn at the interhemispheric fissure and run parallel to the fissure and along the medial aspect of the lateral ventricles. A high-riding third ventricle (between the lateral ventricles) is another typical imaging characteristic. The third ventricle is typically continuous superiorly with the interhemispheric fissure. A CSF collection may be seen in the interhemispheric fissure (cephalad to the high-riding third ventricle) and is referred to as an *interhemispheric cyst*. The cyst may communicate with the third ventricle and one or both of the lateral ventricles. They are often multiloculated and can expand, resulting in compression of the ventricular system and hydrocephalus.

Without the corpus callosum, the cingulate gyri remain everted and the cingulate sulcus does not form. Without the cingulate sulcus, the sulci along the medial aspect of the cerebral hemisphere are seen to radiate outward from the high-riding third ventricle (best seen on the midline sagittal image and demonstrated in this case). These radiating medial hemispheric sulci are the most characteristic imaging finding in corpus callosum agenesis.

SUGGESTED READINGS

Barkovich AJ. Analyzing the corpus callosum. *AJNR* 1996;17:1643–1655.

Barkovich AJ. Apparent atypical callosal dysgenesis: analysis of MR findings in six cases and their relationship to holoprosencephaly. *AJNR* 1990;11:333–339.

Barkovich AJ, Norman D. Anomalies of the corpus callosum: correlation with further anomalies of the brain. *ASNR* 1988;9:493–501.

Curnes JT, Laster DW, Koubek TD, et al. MRI of corpus callosum syndromes. *AJNR* 1986;7:617–622.

Georgy BA, Hesselink JR, Jernigan TL. MR imaging of the corpus callosum. *AJR* 1993;160:949–955.

Mori K. Giant interhemispheric cysts associated with agenesis of the corpus callosum. *J Neurosurg* 1992;76:224–230.

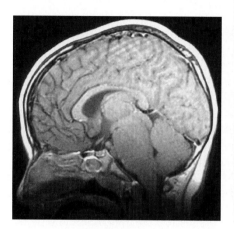

FIGURE 16.1A

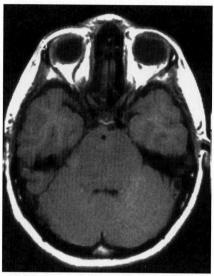

FIGURE 16.1B

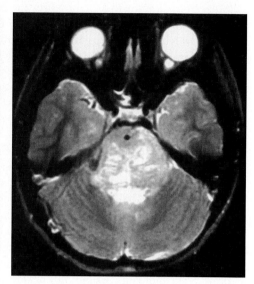

FIGURE 16.1C

CLINICAL HISTORY

A 14-year-old male with multiple cranial neuropathies and ataxia.

FINDINGS

Sagittal T1-weighted acquisition (Fig. 16.1A) demonstrates diffuse enlargement of the brainstem involving the midbrain, pons, and medulla. There is effacement of the normal ventral contour of the brainstem. Axial T1-weighted image (Fig. 16.1B) demonstrates diffuse enlargement of the brainstem with encasement of the basilar artery as well as narrowing of the prepontine cistern. Axial T2-weighted acquisition (Fig. 16.1C) demonstrates heterogeneous high signal throughout the brainstem. There was no significant enhancement following contrast. (Courtesy of George Luh, MD, Loma Linda, California.)

DIAGNOSIS

Brainstem astrocytoma.

DISCUSSION

Brainstem astrocytomas usually occur in children and young adolescents. They account for 10% of all childhood brain tumors. The pons is most commonly involved; however, there is often extension into the medulla, midbrain, and/or cerebellum. Most brainstem astrocytomas are diffuse infiltrative (fibrillary-type) tumors with a high propensity for anaplasia, necrosis, and hemorrhage. Because of their location and infiltrative histology, these tumors are typically not surgically resectable, and irradiation is the primary treatment. Less than 20% of brainstem astrocytomas are histologically benign juvenile pilocytic astrocytomas (JPA), which are bulky, usually dorsally exophytic lesions that have a much better prognosis. The exophytic JPA can occasionally be resected.

A sixth nerve palsy in a child is a typical presenting complaint. Cranial nerve deficits, long tract signs, gait disturbance, and hydrocephalus are all common clinical presentations.

Infiltrative brainstem astrocytoma (seen in this case) appears as an ill-defined hyperintense lesion in the pons on proton density (PD), T2-weighted, and FLAIR images. There may or may not be extension into the upper/lower brainstem or cerebellum. Intratumoral signal is usually heterogeneous, but cyst formation is uncommon. There is typically distortion and enlargement of the pons; an undulating ventral margin of the brainstem (seen on sagittal images) is a characteristic imaging finding. There is often encasement of the basilar artery by tumor and effacement of the prepontine cistern (nicely demonstrated in this case). Contrast enhancement occurs in about one-fourth of cases and is typically focal and nodular when present. Spread of tumor via the subarachnoid space is not uncommon. The prognosis for infiltrative brainstem astrocytoma is poor, with 5-year survival rates of approximately 20%.

In contradistinction to infiltrative lesions, brainstem JPAs are well-circumscribed multicystic masses, which demonstrate intense enhancement. They are dorsally exophytic lesions, which often present as cerebellopontine angle masses.

The differential diagnosis for a brainstem lesion on MRI includes astrocytoma, encephalitis, tuberculoma, demyelinating disease (such as acute disseminated encephalomyelitis, multiple sclerosis, or osmotic demyelination), vascular malformation, and infarction.

SUGGESTED READINGS

Burger PC. Pathology of brainstem astrocytomas. *Pediatr Neurosurg* 1996;24:35–40.

Hoffman HJ. Brainstem gliomas. *Clin Neurosurg* 1997;44:549–558.

Hoffman HJ. Dorsally exophytic brainstem tumors and midbrain tumors. *Pediatr Neurosurg* 1996;24:256–262.

Kane AG, Robles HA, Smirniotopoulos JG, et al. Radiologic-pathologic correlational diffuse pontine astrocytoma. *AJNR* 1993;14:941–945.

Khatib Z, Heidemann R, Kovnar E, et al. Predominance of pilocytic histology in dorsally exophytic brainstem tumors. *Pediatr Neurosurg* 1994;20:2–10.

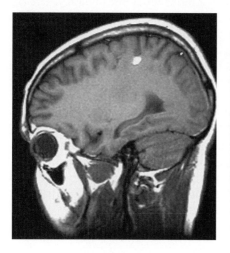

FIGURE 17.1A

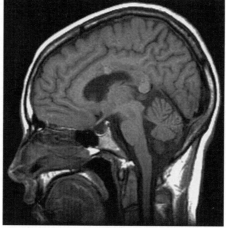

FIGURE 17.1B

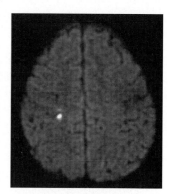

FIGURE 17.1C

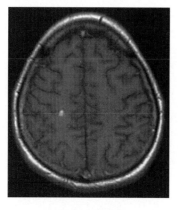

FIGURE 17.1D

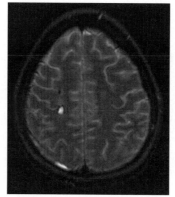

FIGURE 17.1E

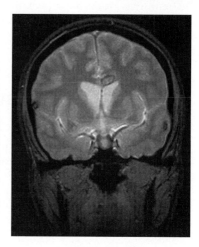

FIGURE 17.1F

CLINICAL HISTORY

34-year-old male involved in a motor vehicle accident.

FINDINGS

Several small scattered foci of abnormal signal intensity are noted at the gray-white junction and body of the corpus callosum. These lesions are bright on T1- and T2-weighted sequences, and demonstrate low signal intensity on the coronal gradient echo sequence, compatible with small hemorrhagic foci (Fig. 17A-F).

DIAGNOSIS

Diffuse axonal injury.

DISCUSSION

Diffuse axonal injury (DAI or shear injury) is seen in patients who suffer severe head trauma and present with profound clinical impairment. There is typically a history of loss of consciousness at the scene. DAI represents nearly half of all primary intraaxial traumatic brain lesions and is the most important cause of significant morbidity in patients sustaining head trauma.

Diffuse axonal injury results from angular or rotational acceleration or deceleration forces of the brain, which lead to multifocal damage to axons, neurons, and blood vessels. Because of the mechanism of injury, DAI is seen most commonly in sites where relatively soft brain is adjacent to more rigid structures within the skull. The most common areas are at the gray-white interface (particularly in a parasagittal location), corpus callosum (specifically involving the body and splenium), and dorsolateral aspect of the upper brainstem (which tends to spare the brainstem surface, as opposed to a direct contusion). Other common sites include the posterior limb of the internal capsule, caudate nuclei, thalamus, and dorsolateral tegmentum.

MRI is the most sensitive imaging modality for evaluation of shearing injury. The majority (approximately 80%) of DAI is hemorrhagic and too small to be detected by CT. The MR signal intensity varies with age of the injury, pulse sequence used, and the presence or absence of hemorrhage. Acute nonhemorrhagic DAI reveals small foci of edema that are hypointense on T1-weighted images and hyperintense on T2-weighted images. After a few days, a central focus of hemorrhage may appear within a previously nonhemorrhagic DAI lesion. This is seen as a punctate focus of hyperintensity on T1-weighted images and hypointensity on T2-weighted images, reflecting the presence of intracellular methemoglobin, which eventually converts to extracellular methemoglobin and follows the typical MR signal characteristics (bright on both T1- and T2-weighted sequences).

Acute hemorrhagic DAI (deoxyhemoglobin) is isointense to adjacent brain on T1-weighted sequences and hypointense to adjacent brain on T2-weighted sequences. Hemorrhagic DAI can be detected by CT as small scattered areas of petechial hemorrhage, and is seen optimally 3–7 days after injury. Gradient echo sequences are the most sensitive in detecting DAI, as deoxyhemoglobin typically blooms on gradient echo imaging. In general, shear injury is best detected 3–7 days after injury and gradually fades over several weeks. However, focal areas of hemosiderin or ferritin may persist indefinitely as decreased signal intensity on T2-weighted sequences. Late sequellae include atrophy and Wallerian degeneration.

Submitted by Elizabeth Vogler, MD, William G. Bradley, MD, PhD (Senior Editor), Long Beach Memorial Medical Center, Long Beach, CA.

SUGGESTED READING

Bradley WG. Hemorrhage. In Stark DD, Bradley WG, eds. *Magnetic Resonance Imaging*, 3rd ed. St. Louis: Mosby, 1999: 1329–1346.

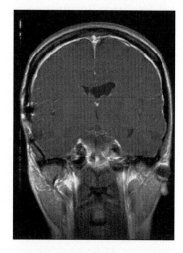

FIGURE 18.1A

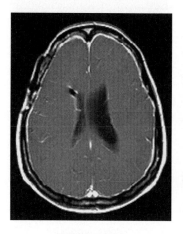

FIGURE 18.1B

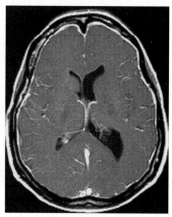

FIGURE 18.1C

CLINICAL HISTORY

A 43-year-old female with a chronic ventriculoperitoneal shunt for communicating hydrocephalus following subarachnoid hemorrhage.

FINDINGS

Diffuse enhancement of the dura is evident on the postcontrast T1-weighted images over the cerebral convexities (Fig. 18.1A–C). The meninges are smooth and thickened. A shunt tube is seen entering the right lateral ventricle (Fig. 18.1B).

DIAGNOSIS

Benign meningeal fibrosis.

DISCUSSION

The association of diffuse meningeal (dural) enhancement with ventriculoperitoneal (VP) shunting was initially described in 1991 by Mokri. The same findings were later documented with other processes that result in meningeal irritation such as repeated lumbar puncture and craniotomy, as well as subarachnoid hemorrhage and intracranial hypotension. The enhancement is benign and may persist for years.

Different hypotheses have been proposed to explain the underlying pathology. Some authorities suggest diffuse pachymeningeal (i.e., dural) fibrosis is associated with long-standing ventricular shunts. This is supported by the fact that meningeal histologic examinations have revealed granulation tissue and marked fibrosis within the subdural space.

The low CSF pressures that have been reported in several cases of this entity secondary to overshunting support the possibility of dural venous dilatation as a possible underlying etiology. Such venous dilatation exerts traction on pain-sensitive structures at the base of the brain, resulting in postural headache. Both the headache and the meningeal enhancement often resolve with shunt revision. These issues remain unsettled because very few studies have been done of shunted patients and because the evidence of meningeal fibrosis is largely drawn from cases of spontaneous intracranial hypotension with subdural fluid collection.

Submitted by Sattam Lingawi, MB, ChB; Peter Brotchie, MBBS, PhD, FRCPC; William G. Bradley, MD, PhD, FACR (Senior Editor), Long Beach Memorial Medical Center, Long Beach, CA.

SUGGESTED READING

Mokri B, Parisi JE, Scheithauer BW, et al. Meningeal biopsy of intracranial hypotension: meningeal enhancement on MRI. *Neurology* 1995;45:1801–1807.

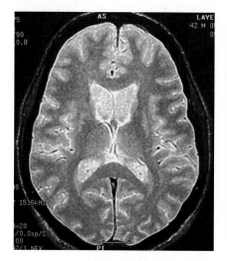

FIGURE 19.1A

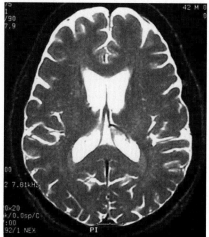

FIGURE 19.1B

CLINICAL HISTORY

A 42-year-old male with a history of choreaform movements.

FINDINGS

Axial proton-density and T2-weighted images (Fig. 19.1A, B) show subtle "squaring-off" of the frontal horns of the lateral ventricles. Note atrophy of the caudate nuclei, best seen on the proton-density acquisition. There is prominence of the ventricles and cortical sulci for a patient 42 years of age, consistent with diffuse cerebral atrophy.

DIAGNOSIS

Huntington's disease.

DISCUSSION

Typically, the diagnosis of Huntington's disease is made clinically, before investigation with MR. Given its hereditary nature (autosomal dominant transmission with full penetrance), each child of an affected patient has a 50% chance of inheriting the disease. Thus although the choreic movements can be associated with a large number of disorders (including infections and Sydenham's chorea, drug-related, and even vascular insults that produce subthalamic nuclear lesions), the presence of family history is key to the diagnosis.

Generally, the movement disorder is followed by progressive onset of dementia and personality disorder. The caudate nucleus and putamen are severely involved with loss of neurons, thus the classic atrophic picture of the corpus striatum. The brain itself develops considerable atrophy in the late stages. Reactive gliosis can be seen in the affected areas. The typical picture of ventricular enlargement in a young patient with marked loss of substance in the caudate nuclei in particular is well shown in this case.

SUGGESTED READING

Starkstein SE, Brandt J, Bylsma F, et al. Neuropsychological correlates of brain atrophy in Huntington's disease: a magnetic resonance imaging study. *Neuroradiology* 1992;34:487–489.

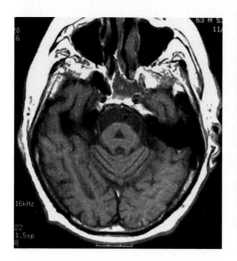

FIGURE 20.1A

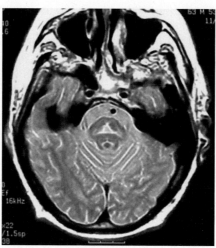

FIGURE 20.1B

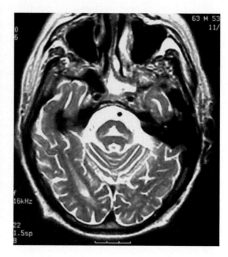

FIGURE 20.1C

CLINICAL HISTORY

A 63-year-old alcoholic male with decreased mental status.

FINDINGS

Axial T1-, proton-density, and T2-weighted images (Fig. 20.1A–C) show a triangular-shaped region of abnormal signal within the pons at the pontomedullary junction. The lesion is hypointense on T1-weighted images and hyperintense on the proton-density and T2-weighted acquisition. There is diffuse cerebral and cerebellar atrophy.

DIAGNOSIS

Central pontine myelinolysis (osmotic myelinolysis).

DISCUSSION

Osmotic myelinolysis (OM) is a toxic demyelinating disease that typically occurs in alcoholic, malnourished, and chronically debilitated patients with severe electrolyte disturbances. Most cases are associated with chronic alcoholism in the setting of rapid correction of hyponatremia. The symptoms of OM are quadraparesis, pseudobulbar palsy, and decreased level of consciousness, often resulting in coma and/or death.

Pathologically, OM is characterized by myelin loss with relative sparing of the neuron. The central pons is the most common site, hence the term *central pontine myelinolysis* (CPM). OM also occurs in extrapontine locations (50% of cases), such as putamina, caudate nuclei, midbrain, thalami, and subcortical white matter (see Case 95).

Nonenhanced CT scans are frequently normal or show subtle hypodensity in the affected areas. On MRI, OM is typically hypointense on T1-weighted images and hyperintense on T2-weighted scans. The characteristic appearance of CPM on PD- and T2-weighted images is a central triangular region of hyperintense signal, simulating a trefoil hat (as seen in this case). This pattern reflects the propensity of OM to most severely affect the central transverse fibers, with characteristic sparing of the descending corticospinal tracts, the peripheral pial and ventricular surface rim of tissue. Enhancement is uncommon but can occur most frequently at the periphery of the lesion.

Extrapontine myelinolysis can occur without the presence of pontine disease. Temporal studies have shown that MRI findings lag behind clinical signs of improvement. Lesions may not completely resolve despite clinical recovery.

The differential diagnosis for nonenhancing high signal in the pons includes infarct, glioma, multiple sclerosis, progressive multifocal leukoencephalopathy, rhombencephalitis, and radiation or chemotherapy change. If there is abnormal signal within the basal ganglia as well, the findings are more specific for osmotic myelinolysis. Differential diagnosis would still include hypoxia, Leigh disease (see Vol. 1, Case 90), and Wilson disease.

SUGGESTED READINGS

Hadfield MG, Kubal WS. Extrapontine myelinolysis of the basal ganglia without central pontine myelinolysis. *Clin Neuropathol* 1996;15:96–100.

Huin E, Tan KP. CT and MR findings in central pontine and extrapontine myelinolysis—a study of two patients. *Singapore Med J* 1996;37:622–666.

Laubenberger J, Schneider B, Ansorge O, et al. Central pontine myelinolysis: clinical presentation and radiologic findings. *Eur Radiol* 1996;6:177–183.

Miller GM, Baker HL Jr, Okozaki H, et al. Central pontine myelinolysis and its imitators: MR findings. *Radiology* 1988;168:795–802.

Valk J, van der Knaap MS. Toxic encephalopathy. *AJNR* 1992;13:747–760.

Yuh WT, Simonson TM, D'Alessandro MP, et al. Temporal changes of MR findings in central pontine myelinolysis. *AJNR* 1995;16[Suppl]:975–977.

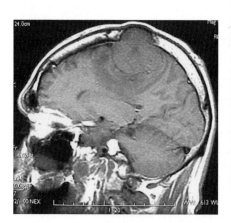

FIGURE 21.1A

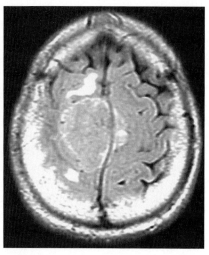

FIGURE 21.1B

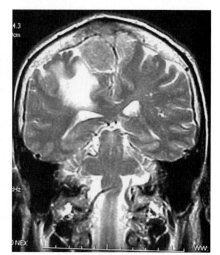

FIGURE 21.1C

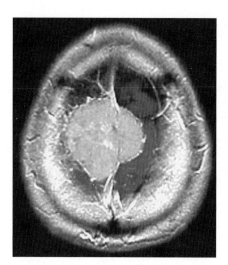

FIGURE 21.1D

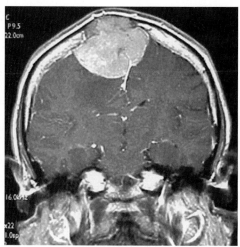

FIGURE 21.1E

CLINICAL HISTORY

A 50-year-old male describes a "lump" on the top of his head.

FINDINGS

Sagittal noncontrast T1-weighted acquisition (Fig. 21.1A) demonstrates a large extraaxial mass. There is a broad base of dural attachment along the inner table of the calvarium. Underlying cortex is displaced. There is surrounding low intensity within the subjacent brain parenchyma consistent with edema. The mass is well defined and has eroded through both the inner and outer tables of the overlying calvarium, producing a soft-tissue mass within the scalp. Note widening of the subarachnoid space ventral to this mass, suggestive of an extraaxial lesion. Axial FLAIR and coronal T2-weighted images (Fig. 21.1B,C) show the mass as interme-diate in signal with significant perilesional edema, and shift of the midline structures to the left. There is extension along both sides of the interhemispheric falx. Postcontrast T1-weighted images (Fig. 21.1D,E) show a well-defined, intensely enhancing mass. Note extension of the tumor into the region of the superior sagittal sinus on the coronal image. There is no enhancement of the sinus suggestive of occlusion. Coronal T2-weighted image demonstrates a triangular-shaped focus of intermediate signal material within the superior sagittal sinus at the level of the mass, consistent with tumor invasion and/or thrombosis.

DIAGNOSIS

Meningioma with destruction of overlying calvarium and thrombosis of the superior sagittal sinus.

DISCUSSION

Meningiomas are the most common primary nonglial intracranial tumor. They are most commonly found in middle-aged and older people. There is a female predominance of 2:1 in the adult population. Meningiomas are rare in the pediatric population and when present are frequently associated with neurofibromatosis. The possibility of neurofibromatosis should be considered in any patient with multiple meningiomas. Meningiomas coexist in patients with breast carcinoma and can arise several years after irradiation, "radiation-induced" meningioma.

Meningiomas arise from the meninges or cell rests of meningeal derivation. They have a predilection for areas associated with arachnoid granulations and are most often found along the convexity attached to the sagittal sinus. Other favorite areas include the dura adjacent to the anterior Sylvian fissure, the sphenoid wing, tuberculum sellae, perisellar region, and olfactory grooves. In the posterior fossa they tend to arise along the petrous bone in the cerebellopontine angle, the clivus, along the tentorial leaf, and at the free edge of the tentorium. Meningiomas usually have a broad base of dural attachment but can occasionally arise without dural attachment within the Sylvian fissure or ventricles. The lateral ventricle is the most commonly involved followed by the third and fourth ventricles.

The first and most important step in the diagnosis of meningioma is to determine if the tumor is extraaxial. There are several criteria to help make this decision. A broad-based dural attachment is strongly suggestive but not definitive. Bony hyperostosis and/or calvarial invasion are highly specific for extraaxial origin. The other highly specific sign is the visualization of pial vascular structures, cerebrospinal fluid (CSF) clefts, and dural margins between the tumor and cerebral cortex. Pial blood vessel interfaces appear as punctate and curvilinear signal voids on all pulse sequences at the junction of the tumor with underlying brain. The vascular structures may be arteries or veins. About 80% of meningiomas will demonstrate a vascular margin at the interface with the brain. Eighty percent of meningiomas will also demonstrate a CSF cleft between the tumor and underlying brain parenchyma. The dural margin interface is seen primarily in meningiomas of the cavernous sinus. It appears as a low-intensity rim on all pulse sequences separating the tumor from the adjacent temporal lobe. Often, however, the tumor can be seen to invade directly through the dura and abut the adjacent brain. Meningiomas along the falx and tentorium, as in this case, can also invade through the dura to its opposite side. It is important to note that intraaxial tumors almost never invade the dura unless there has been previous surgery. Metastases can occasionally grow exophytically from brain parenchyma and invade dura; however, there will be no tumor/brain interface.

Another valuable tool in determining if a mass is extraaxial is the buckling of the cortical gyri subjacent to the extraaxial mass into an onion-skin-like configuration beginning at the margin of the tumor (shown in this case). This sign is better seen on MRI and with large meningiomas.

On unenhanced CT, meningiomas are usually slightly hyperdense. The tumor is calcified in approximately 20% of cases. Rarely, meningiomas show cystic, osteoblastic, chondromatous, or fatty degeneration. On MRI, the typical signal characteristics consist of iso- to slightly hypointense signal relative to gray matter on T1-weighted images and range from hypo- to hyperintense signal relative to gray matter on T2-weighted images. There is characteristically intense homogeneous enhancement of meningiomas. Occasionally, they have necrotic centers, which may not enhance. The dural tail, a crescentic tail of enhancement at the tumor/dura interface, is typically seen with meningioma, although it is not specific. Dural metastases and occasionally schwannomas can show this uncommonly. The degree of parenchymal edema within subjacent brain is variable, but the slow growth of the tumor produces brain atrophy; thus little mass effect may be seen with large lesions. Rarely, meningiomas invade underlying brain parenchyma.

Meningioma can also grow in an "en plaque" fashion, appearing as a region of diffuse dural thickening. Differentiation from dural metastasis, lymphoma, and sarcoidosis can be difficult.

Meningiomas may encase and narrow adjacent vessels, most notably when they occur in the parasellar region. (See Vol. 2, Case 34.) Adjacent dural venous sinuses can be invaded and/or occluded (as seen in this case). Bony changes associated with meningiomas may be hyperostotic or osteolytic. Meningioma can even invade through the calvarium and present as a scalp mass (shown in this case). Sphenoid or ethmoid sinus expansion can be seen with adjacent meningioma.

Complete surgical excision is the treatment of choice. A recent study described more frequent recurrence of lobulated or "mushrooming" meningiomas as compared with rounded tumors. These tumors therefore require a more aggressive surgical approach with wider surgical margins. Important preoperative imaging issues for meningioma include invasion of underlying parenchyma, invasion of the cavernous sinus, compression or invasion of the dural venous sinuses, and/or the presence of vascular encasement.

SUGGESTED READINGS

Elster AD, Challa VR, Gilbert TH, et al. Meningioma: MR and histopathological features. *Radiology* 1989;170:857–862.

Goldberg HI, Lavi E, Atlas SW. Extra-axial brain tumors. In: Atlas SW, ed. *Magnetic resonance imaging of the brain and spine*, 2nd ed. Philadelphia: Lippincott-Raven, 1996:424–446.

Goldsher D, Litt AW, Pinto RS, et al. Dural "tail" associated with meningiomas on Gd-DTPA-enhanced MR images: characteristics, differential diagnostic value, and possible implications for treatment. *Radiology* 1990;176:447–450.

Nakasu S, Nakasu Y, Nakajima M, et al. Preoperative identification of meningiomas that are highly likely to recur. *J Neurosurg* 1999;90:455–462.

Osborn AG. Meningiomas and other nonglial neoplasms. In: *Diagnostic neuroradiology.* St. Louis: Mosby, 1994:584–601.

Wasenko JJ, Hochhauser L, Stopa EG, Winfield JA. Cystic meningioma: MR characteristics and surgical correlation. *AJNR* 1994;15:1959–1965.

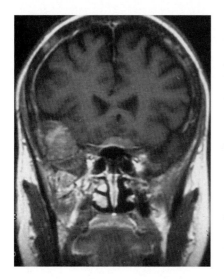

FIGURE 22.1A

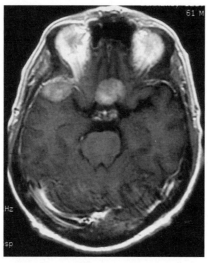

FIGURE 22.1B

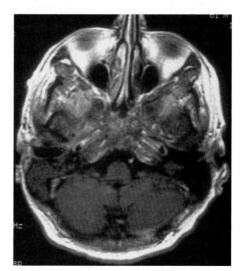

FIGURE 22.1C

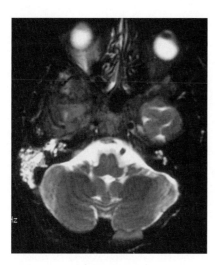

FIGURE 22.1D

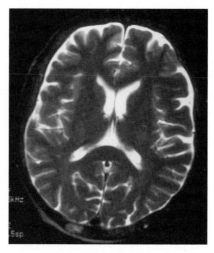

FIGURE 22.1E

CLINICAL HISTORY

A 61-year-old male with known prostate carcinoma now with decreasing vision in the left eye and right hearing loss.

FINDINGS

Multiple bony and dural-based lesions are noted, compressing the left optic canal (Fig. 22.1A,B) and right Eustachian tube (Fig. 22.1C,D).

DIAGNOSIS

Bony and dural metastases.

DISCUSSION

Prostate carcinoma is one of the few cancers that metastasizes directly to the dura, potentially simulating meningiomas. In this case, both dural metastases and bony metastases are seen. Since prostate carcinoma has a relatively low water content and high nuclear/cytoplasmic ratio, the metastases appear dark on T2-weighted images (Fig. 22.1D,E).

The decreasing left visual acuity can be explained by compromise of the left optic canal (Fig. 22.1A). A metastasis to the dura of the planum sphenoidale has caused somewhat greater compression of the left optic canal than the right. Metastatic disease to the skull base (Fig. 22.1C) has compressed the right Eustachian tube, leading to fluid backup in the middle ear and mastoid (Fig. 22.1D), decreasing hearing.

Bony metastases explain the mottled appearance of the marrow space. The metastases tend to enhance with contrast and to appear relatively bright on T2-weighted images (Fig. 22.1D,E).

Submitted by William G. Bradley, MD, PhD, FACR (Senior Editor), Long Beach Memorial Medical Center, Long Beach, CA.

SUGGESTED READING

Atlas SW. Orbit. In: Stark DD, Bradley WG, eds. *Magnetic resonance imaging*, 3rd ed. St. Louis: Mosby, 1999:1637–1666.

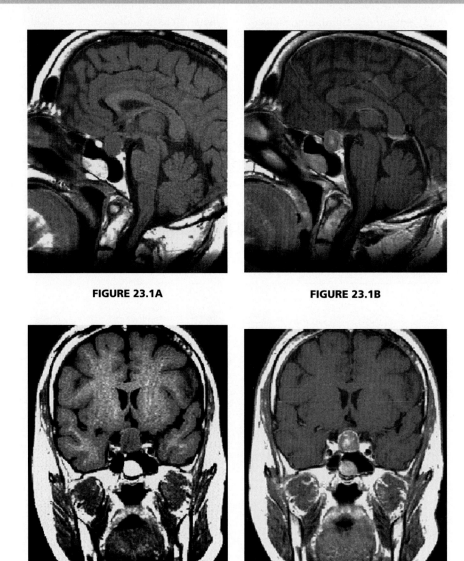

FIGURE 23.1A

FIGURE 23.1B

FIGURE 23.1C

FIGURE 23.1D

CLINICAL HISTORY

A 38-year-old male with bitemporal hemianopsia.

FINDINGS

A 2-cm mass expands the pituitary fossa with supratentorial extension and compression of the optic chiasm. The mass is hypointense on T1-weighted images (Fig. 23.1A,C) and enhances heterogeneously with contrast (Fig. 23.1B,D).

DIAGNOSIS

Pituitary macroadenoma.

DISCUSSION

Pituitary macroadenomas are benign tumors of the pituitary gland that measure more than 10 mm. These tumors are usually hormonally inactive. The most common hormonally active macroadenomas are prolactinomas. Patients usually present with visual disturbance (i.e., bitemporal hemianopsia). In addition, women may present with galactorrhea and men may present with loss of libido.

Although CT has played an important historical role in pituitary imaging, MRI is now considered the preferable modality because of its superior soft-tissue contrast. Although gadolinium is required for microadenomas, nonenhanced MRI is sufficient for macroadenomas. This is primarily due to the large size of the tumor and the natural contrast against the surrounding CSF. MR protocols include coronal, sagittal, and occasionally axial images that are needed to differentiate the tumor from adjacent vital structures such as the optic chiasm, the hypothalamus, and the floor of the third ventricle. Accurate evaluation of involvement of the cavernous sinuses is often difficult because they have a similar pattern of enhancement to the tumor itself and the medial dural reflection is poorly visualized. In cases with cavernous sinus invasion, the prolactin level is usually very high (more than 1,000 ng/ml).

The tumor is usually isointense to brain parenchyma and enhances heterogeneously due to the cystic changes, necrosis, and intratumoral hemorrhage, which are common. As the tumor enlarges it compresses the optic chiasm above (leading to bitemporal hemianopsia) and the residual normal pituitary tissue below (leading to pituitary insufficiency).

The differential diagnosis in the setting of hormonal activity is virtually nonexistent. However, without hormonal abnormalities, suprasellar aneurysms, hypothalamic gliomas, meningiomas, craniopharyngiomas, and pituitary metastases must be considered.

Submitted by Sattam Lingawi, MB, ChB; Peter Brotchie, MBBS, PhD, FRCPC; William G. Bradley, MD, PhD, FACR (Senior Editor), Long Beach Memorial Medical Center, Long Beach, CA.

SUGGESTED READINGS

Davis PC, Gokhale KA, Joseph GJ, et al. Pituitary adenoma: correlation of half-dose gadolinium-enhanced MR imaging with surgical findings in 26 patients. *Radiology* 1991;180:779.
Kucharczyk W, Davis DO, Kelly WM, et al. Pituitary adenomas: high-resolution MR imaging at 1.5 T. *Radiology* 1986;161:761.
Lundin P, Bergstrom K. Gd-DTPA-enhanced MR imaging of pituitary macroadenomas. *Acta Radiol* 1992;33:323.
Scotti G, Yu CY, Dillon WP, et al. MR imaging of cavernous sinus involvement by pituitary adenomas. *AJR* 1988;151:799.

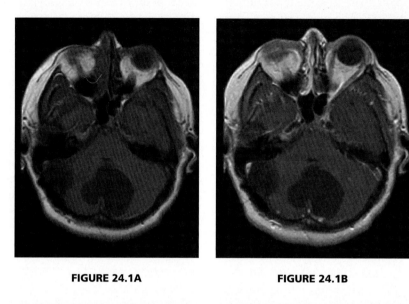

FIGURE 24.1A   **FIGURE 24.1B**

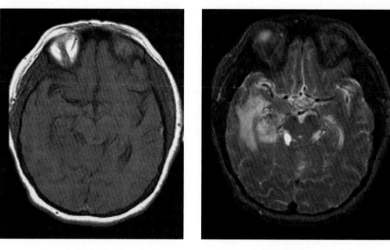

FIGURE 24.1C   **FIGURE 24.1D**

CLINICAL HISTORY

A 39-year-old female with craniotomy for brain tumor resection several years ago now complains of difficulty walking.

FINDINGS

T1-weighted images demonstrate a large cystic lesion in the cerebellum (Fig. 24.1A) with an enhancing mural nodule (Fig. 24.1B). A second solid lesion was evident in the right temporal lobe (Fig. 24.1C,D).

DIAGNOSIS

Supra- and infratentorial hemangioblastomas in Von-Hippel Lindau (VHL).

DISCUSSION

VHL is an autosomal dominant disorder with incomplete penetrance that has variable expression. VHL patients commonly become symptomatic in their 30s or earlier if retinal angiomas or hemangioblastomas of the brain and spinal cord develop.

VHL is a multisystem disease that is characterized by cysts, angiomas, and neoplasms of the CNS and abdominal viscera. Common lesions are cerebellar and spinal hemangioblastomas (accounting for 75% and 25% of all VHL hemangioblastomas, respectively), retinal angiomas (in 40% to 50% of VHL cases), and visceral neoplasia (especially renal cell carcinoma). Cysts within the kidneys, pancreas, and spleen occur in 50% of cases.

The clinical diagnosis of VHL for patients with an affected first-order family member can be made in the presence of one CNS or one visceral manifestation. In the absence of a family history, the diagnosis is made by the presence of multiple hemangioblastomas of the CNS or the coexistence of a single CNS hemangioblastoma and a visceral manifestation.

Submitted by Peter Brotchie, MBBS, PhD; Sattam Lingawi, MB, ChB, FRCPC; William G. Bradley, MD, PhD, FACR (Senior Editor), Long Beach Memorial Medical Center, Long Beach, CA.

SUGGESTED READING

Choyke PL, Glenn GM, Walther MM, et al. Von Hippel-Lindau disease: genetics, clinical and imaging features. *Radiology* 1995;194:629–642.

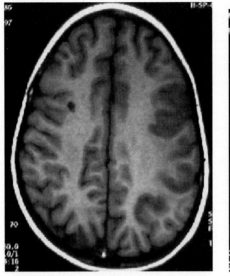

FIGURE 25.1A   **FIGURE 25.1B**

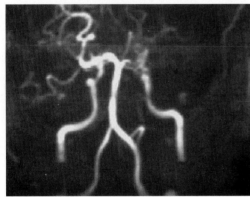
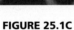
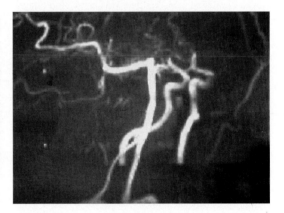

FIGURE 25.1C   **FIGURE 25.1D**

CLINICAL HISTORY

A 19-year-old male with a history of migraine who presented with aphasia, right upper-extremity weakness, and lethargy.

FINDINGS

Low signal on the T1-weighted image (Fig. 25.1A) and high signal on the T2-weighted image (Fig. 25.1B) are noted in a gyriform pattern in the left middle cerebral artery (MCA) territory consistent with cerebral infarction. MRA shows occlusion of the left posterior cerebral artery (PCA) and of both internal carotid arteries (ICAs) with small vessels arising from the occluded segments giving a "puff of smoke" appearance.

DIAGNOSIS

Idiopathic progressive arteriopathy (moyamoya).

DISCUSSION

Moyamoya disease is an idiopathic pathologic condition characterized by progressive narrowing of the supraclinoid ICAs and an abnormal vascular network, known as moyamoya vessels, at the base of the brain.

The imaging findings in moyamoya disease may be classified as primary or secondary. The primary findings are essentially the changes occurring in vessels. Although angiography plays a major role in diagnosing and staging this entity, MRI and MRA guidelines for diagnosis have been developed. These include bilateral stenosis or occlusion of terminal ICAs, anterior cerebral artery (ACA), and MCA on MRA; abnormal vascular network in the basal ganglia on MRA; and greater than two flow voids in the basal ganglia on MRI.

The secondary brain findings include cerebral infarction, white matter disease, atrophy, and hemorrhage. The infarctions have a distinct distribution. They are unevenly distributed in the cortical and subcortical areas of the middle-ACA and middle-PCA border zones. They are less frequently seen in the basal ganglia and thalami. Hemorrhage may occur from aneurysms developing in the abnormal perforator arteries.

Different surgical procedures are used to manage this disease. Anastomosis of the superficial temporal artery to the middle cerebral artery is the most common procedure. (This procedure is usually more successful in children than in adults.)

Submitted by Peter Brotchie, MBBS, PhD; Sattam Lingawi, MB, ChB, FRCPC; William G. Bradley, MD, PhD, FACR (Senior Editor), Long Beach Memorial Medical Center, Long Beach, CA.

SUGGESTED READING

Hasuo K, Mihm F, Matsushima T. MRI and MR angiography in moyamoya disease. *JMRI* 1998;8:762–766.

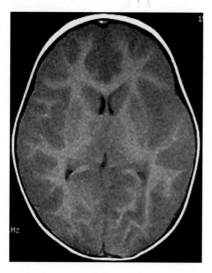

FIGURE 26.1A

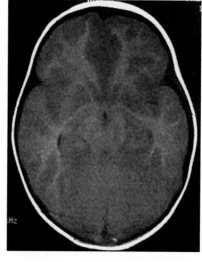

FIGURE 26.1B

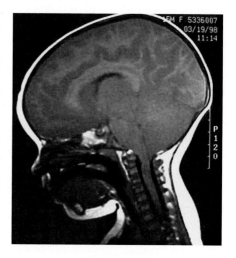

FIGURE 26.1C

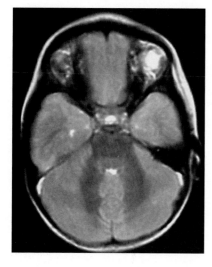

FIGURE 26.1D

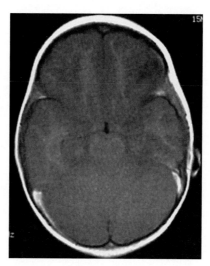

FIGURE 26.1E

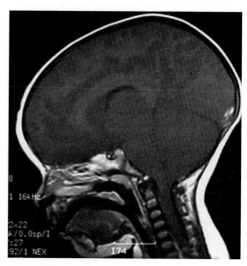

FIGURE 26.1F

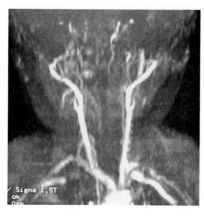

FIGURE 26.1G

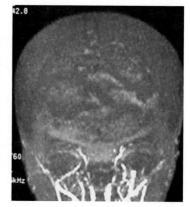

FIGURE 26.1H

CLINICAL HISTORY

A 15-month-old female with history of dehydration suffered a respiratory arrest and is now unresponsive to stimuli.

FINDINGS

Axial T1- and T2-weighted images (Fig. 26.1A,B) show diffuse thickening of the cortical gray matter. The ventricles are slitlike in configuration. Note obliteration of the basal cisterns. No cortical sulci are identified. Differentiation of gray and white matter is obscured in the posterior fossa on the T1-weighted acquisition. Sagittal T1-weighted image (Fig. 26.1C) shows marked swelling of the cerebellar hemispheres with inferior displacement of the cerebellar tonsils through the foramen magnum as well as superior herniation of the cerebellum through the tentorial hiatus. Axial T2-weighted image (Fig. 26.1D) shows flow void within the basilar artery but loss of signal void in the cavernous internal carotid arteries. Axial and sagittal postcontrast T1-weighted images (Fig. 26.1E,F) show no enhancement of the normally enhancing intracranial structures (i.e., circle of Willis, pituitary, or dura). Two-dimensional time-of-flight MRA of the neck and three-dimensional time-of-flight MRA of the intracranial vessels (Fig. 26.1G,H)) show abrupt termination of flow within the ICAs at the skull base. There is no arterial flow identified within the brain.

DIAGNOSIS

Diffuse cerebral edema with brain death, consequent to anoxic insult.

DISCUSSION

Brain death is typically a clinical diagnosis, confirmed with radionuclide cerebral blood flow studies or conventional catheter angiography. More recently, the utility of MRI and MRA as reliable noninvasive imaging modalities in the diagnosis of brain death has been advocated.

The absence of cerebral blood flow is generally accepted as a sign of brain death. Brain death is usually the result of a severe traumatic or anoxic injury. Although the exact pathophysiology of the cessation of blood flow in brain death is not fully understood, the increased intracranial pressure that results from diffuse cerebral edema is thought to be the primary cause.

At imaging, there is diffuse swelling of the cerebral gyri and cerebellar cortex with loss of the subarachnoid space, "slitlike" ventricles, and obliteration of the basal cisterns, as seen in this case. The lack of CSF surrounding the brain can give the brain a "supernormal" appearance. There is typically prolongation of T1 and T2 signal in the involved gyri and deep gray matter nuclei. Transentorial and tonsillar herniations are usually present. These findings alone, however, should not be considered indicative of brain death since they can be observed in patients with severe hypoxic-ischemic injury without brain death.

Orrison et al. identified six common MRI findings in the setting of brain death: transtentorial and tonsillar herniation, absent flow void within the intracranial arteries, poor gray/white matter differentiation, no intracranial enhancement, carotid artery enhancement (intravascular enhancement sign), and prominent nasal and scalp enhancement (MR hot nose sign).

MRA findings in brain death are more specific. Findings include lack of flow within the ICAs above the supraclinoid portion of the vessel and absence of the intracranial branches (nicely demonstrated in this case).

SUGGESTED READINGS

Aichner F, Felber S, Birbamer G, et al. Magnetic resonance: a noninvasive approach to metabolism, circulation, and morphology in human brain death. *Ann Neurol* 1992;32:507–511.

Ishii K, Ohuma T, Kinoshita T, et al. Brain death: MR and MR angiography. *AJNR* 1996;17:731–735.

Matsumura A, Meguro K, Tsurushima H, et al. MRI of brain death. *Neurol Med Chir (Tokyo)* 1996;36:166–171.

Orrison WW Jr, Champlin AM, Kesterson OL, et al. MR "hot nose sign" and "intravascular enhancement sign." *AJNR* 1994;15:913–916.

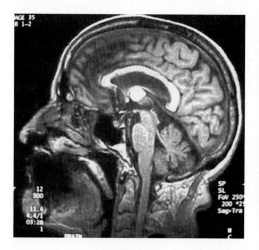

FIGURE 27.1A

FIGURE 27.1B

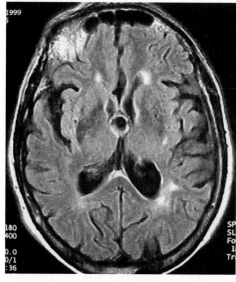
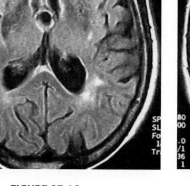

FIGURE 27.1C

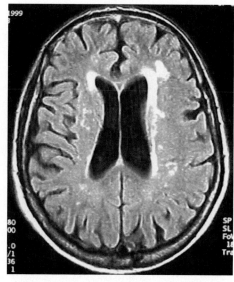

FIGURE 27.1D

CLINICAL HISTORY

A 75-year-old female with history of positional headache.

FINDINGS

Sagittal, noncontrast T1-weighted acquisition (Fig. 27.1A) demonstrates a well-defined rounded high-signal mass within the anterior superior aspect of the third ventricle. Axial T2-weighted (Fig. 27.1B) and FLAIR acquisitions (Fig. 27.1C,D) demonstrate hypointense signal centrally within the lesion. Note the position of the lesion between the lateral fornices. There is mild dilation of the lateral ventricles with apparent transependymal accumulation of cerebral spinal fluid suggestive of obstruction at the level of the foramen of Monro. Incidentally noted are several foci of deep white matter ischemic change.

DIAGNOSIS

Colloid cyst.

DISCUSSION

Colloid cysts are rare benign neoplasms classified as a type of neuroepithelial cyst, similar in histolog to choroid plexus and pineal cysts. More recent studies, however, suggest that colloid cysts are actually derived from endoderm. Radiographically, there is support for this contention in that colloid cysts demonstrate variable density and signal characteristics, whereas choroid plexus and pineal cysts are usually isointense to cerebrospinal fluid (CSF).

Although pathoogically benign, colloid cysts are important to identify because of their association with sudden death due to acute obstruction of the lateral ventricles at the level of the foramen of Monro based on their unique location, situated within the anterior and superior aspect of the third ventricle, between the columns of the fornix. In most cases, the patients are asymptomatic. The most frequent presenting complaint is intermittent headache, often associated with visual changes.

The cysts are iso- to hyperdense on CT. Signal characteristics are highly variable on MRI. The most common appearance is a well-defined hyperintense mass on T1-weighted images that is hypointense on T2-weighted acquisition. There can be subtle peripheral enhancement. Subtle thickening of the septum pellucidum at the level of the foramen of Monro may be the only abnormality on noncontrast MRI. The best approach, if there is high clinical suspicion, is to look for the mass on the sagittal T1-weighted images, superior and posterior to the anterior commissure. Gadolinium may help to better delineate small lesions.

Several theories in the literature today try to explain the characteristic density and signal characteristics of colloid cysts on CT and MRI. Cholesterol crystals, calcium, copper, silicon, and magnesium have all been suggested. Paramagnetic ions were thought to account for the hypointensity on T2-weighted images, but several recent studies have shown that iron content is actually low.

There appears to be no correlation between the size of the colloid cyst and the presence or absence of symptoms. Studies suggest that asymptomatic colloid cysts can be safely managed with observation and serial neuroimaging. Neurosurgical intervention is only necessary if the patient becomes symptomatic, the cyst enlarges, or hydrocephalus develops. Stereotactic cyst aspiration and surgical excision via a transcallosal approach are the two primary treatment options available today. In an experienced surgeon's hands, surgical excision has relatively low morbidity and portends a better long-term outcome due to a lower recurrence rate, as opposed to cyst aspiration.

Differential diagnostic considerations for third ventricular mass include glioma, ependymoma (or subependymoma), giant cell astrocytoma, meningioma, granuloma, choroid plexus neoplasm, and aneurysm. CSF flow artifact in the third ventricle can mimic colloid cyst.

SUGGESTED READINGS

Mamourian AC, Cromwell LD, Harbaugh RE. Colloid cysts of the third ventricle: sometimes more conspicuous on CT than MR. *AJNR* 1998;19:875–878.

Mathiesen T, Grane P, Lindgren L, et al. Third ventricle colloid cysts: a consecutive 12-year series. *J Neurosurg* 1997;86:5–12.

Pollock BE, Huston J 3rd. Natural history of asymptomatic colloid cysts of the third ventricle. *J Neurosurg* 1999;91:364–369.

Veerman EC, Go KG, Molenaar WM, et al. On the chemical characterization of colloid cyst contents. *Acta Neurochir* 1998;140;303–306.

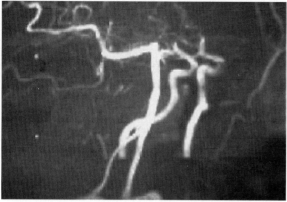

FIGURE 28.1A

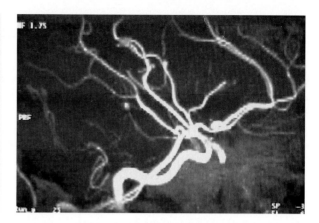

FIGURE 28.1B

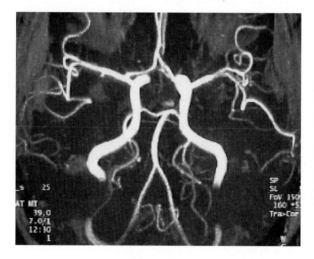

FIGURE 28.1C

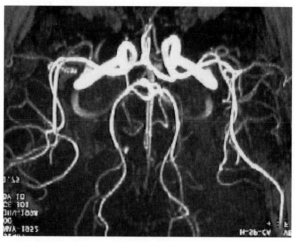

FIGURE 28.1D

CLINICAL HISTORY

A 25-year-old male with a family history of polycystic kidney disease.

FINDINGS

Three-dimensional time-of-flight MR angiogram shows a small 2-mm rounded structure arising from the right posterior cerebral artery (Fig. 28.1A–D).

DIAGNOSIS

Posterior cerebral artery aneurysm.

DISCUSSION

MRA in the brain is most commonly performed using time-of-flight (TOF) techniques. The TOF techniques use flow-related enhancement as the basis of angiotomography. This is best acquired using a short TR gradient-echo sequence with a small flip angle. The images can be acquired by obtaining multiple single slices (two-dimensional [2D] TOF) or slabs of tissue (three-dimensional TOF). The 2D slices should be acquired in the direction countercurrent to the flow in the vessels (i.e., acquired top-to-bottom for arteries and bottom-to-top for veins). The source images are stacked together and a maximum-intensity-projection (MIP) algorithm is used to form an angiogram, which can be viewed from any angle. When the area of coverage is larger than 6 cm, a multiple overlapping thin-section acquisition (MOTSA) is often used to increase coverage and maintain the high resolution of the 3D TOF technique.

Because of its noninvasive nature, MRA is being increasingly used for the assessment of intracranial and extracranial atherosclerotic changes and aneurysms. For aneurysms more than 2 mm, MRA has high sensitivity (87%), specificity (88%), and positive predictive value (99%). The figures are somewhat lower for vessels that are less than 1 mm in diameter (e.g., posterior and anterior communicating arteries). In general, the source images are more sensitive than the computer-generated MIP images.

Submitted by Sattam Lingawi, MB, ChB, FRCPC; Peter Brotchie, MBBS, PhD; William G. Bradley, MD, PhD, FACR (Senior Editor), Long Beach Memorial Medical Center, Long Beach, CA.

SUGGESTED READINGS

Stock KW, Wetzel S, Kirsch E, et al. Anatomic evaluation of the circle of Willis: MR angiography versus intra-arterial digital subtraction angiography. *AJNR* 1996;17:1495–1499.

Whittemore AR, Bradley WG, Jinkins JR. Comparison of cocurrent and countercurrent flow-related enhancement in MR imaging. *Radiology* 1989;170:265–271.

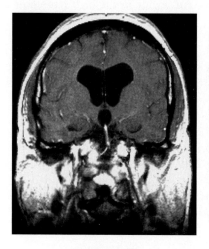

FIGURE 29.1A

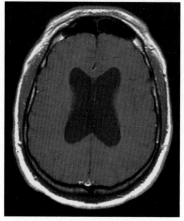

FIGURE 29.1B

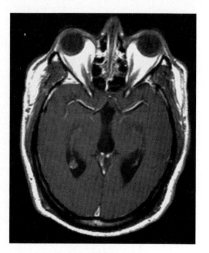

FIGURE 29.1C

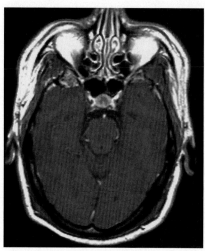

FIGURE 29.1D

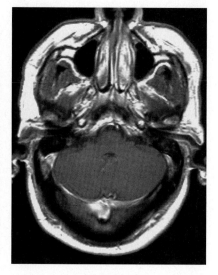

FIGURE 29.1E

CLINICAL HISTORY

A 37-year-old male with uncontrollable headaches.

FINDINGS

There is moderate dilatation of the third and lateral ventricles (Fig. 29.1A–C) with sparing of the fourth ventricle (Fig. 29.1D) and a small aqueduct of Sylvius (Fig. 29.1A–E).

DIAGNOSIS

Aqueductal stenosis.

DISCUSSION

Obstruction of the aqueduct of Sylvius may be related to congenital, inflammatory, or neoplastic processes. The most common cause of aqueductal occlusion is gliosis as the result of subarachnoid hemorrhage or infection. Congenital causes include aqueductal stenosis secondary to atresia, webs, or fenestrations, which may be seen in isolation or in association with other congenital disorders, such as the Chiari malformations. Inflammatory causes include lesions arising within the aqueduct or in the periaqueductal tissues, such as inflammation from acute demyelinating plaques or brainstem encephalitis. Neoplastic causes include brainstem tumors, particularly tectal gliomas, third ventricular tumors that grow posteriorly, or pineal tumors that grow forward, compressing the tectum and aqueduct. Acute obstruction of the aqueduct can be caused by hemorrhage or migration of a cysticercal cyst.

Most patients with congenital aqueductal stenosis present *in utero* or as neonates. In some cases, a pinhole in the membrane may allow enough CSF flow through the aqueduct to prevent symptoms. Presentation is delayed until childhood or even into the patient's 30s (particularly in young women), most likely related to the increased produc-

tion of CSF. In cases where an obstructing membrane is implicated, surgical perforation can be a successful treatment. However, in most instances, the specific type of anatomic obstruction (atresia, web, or fenestration) is not resolvable with imaging, and most patients who present with aqueductal stenosis are shunted.

The radiographic findings in aqueductal stenosis are dilatation of the third and lateral ventricles, with a small aqueduct and sparing of the fourth ventricle. MRI is the imaging modality of choice, because of its ability to acquire thin slices directly in the sagittal plane, thereby increasing sensitivity to such anatomic considerations or to small periaqueductal masses. Additionally, aqueductal patency can be assessed by evaluating the flow void created by the normal pulsatile flow of CSF back and forth through the aqueduct. With aqueductal stenosis, flow through the aqueduct is diminished and the flow void is not seen. (Note: Use of gradient-moment nulling ["flow compensation"] may result in rephasing of CSF flow, decreasing the sensitivity of the flow void as a sign of aqueductal patency. Alternatively, single-slice gradient-echo imaging increases flow-related enhancement, resulting in increased sensitivity to flow.)

Submitted by Elizabeth Vogler, MD; Alan Chan, MD; William G. Bradley, MD, PhD, FACR (Senior Editor), Long Beach Memorial Medical Center, Long Beach, CA.

SUGGESTED READING

Bradley WG, Quencer RM. Hydrocephalus and cerebrospinal fluid flow. In: Stark DD, Bradley WG, eds. *Magnetic resonance imaging,* 3rd ed. St. Louis: Mosby, 1999:1483–1508.

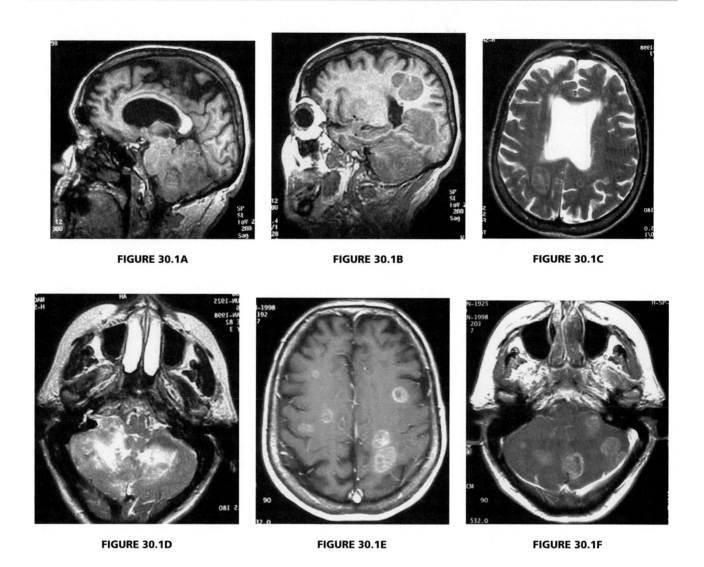

FIGURE 30.1A **FIGURE 30.1B** **FIGURE 30.1C**

FIGURE 30.1D **FIGURE 30.1E** **FIGURE 30.1F**

CLINICAL HISTORY

A 78-year-old female with recent change in mental status.

FINDINGS

Sagittal T1-weighted image (Fig. 30.1A,B) demonstrates multiple, large, well-defined regions of hypointense signal within the subcortical white matter of the cerebral hemispheres and within the posterior fossa. Axial T2-weighted acquisition (Fig. 30.1C,D) demonstrates multiple, corresponding, subtly hyperintense lesions. Following intravenous contrast, T1-weighted images (Fig. 30.1E,F) show multiple ring-enhancing lesions throughout the supratentorial and infratentorial brain parenchyma, predominantly located at the corticomedullary junction.

DIAGNOSIS

Ovarian metastases.

DISCUSSION

Metastatic tumor to the brain typically occurs via hematogenous spread of tumor from an extracranial site, or occasionally by direct extension from skull metastases or nasopharyngeal routes. Hematogenous metastases may deposit in the brain parenchyma, dura, or calvarium. The primary tumors that most frequently metastasize to the brain are lung, breast, skin (melanoma), gastrointestinal, and genitourinary neoplasms. In adults, cerebral metastases are common, representing 25% to 35% of all brain tumors. In more than 80% of cases, parenchymal metastases are multifocal; however, solitary metastases do occur (30% to 50%), usually from lung, breast, or melanoma primaries. All areas of the brain can be affected, but the corticomedullary junction is the most common site. This is related to the dramatic narrowing of the diameter of the arterioles that supply the cortex in this region. Less than 20% of metastases are hemorrhagic; these include choriocarcinoma, renal cell carcinoma, melanoma, and thyroid carcinomas.

Clinically, parenchymal metastases range from asymptomatic (usually lung cancer or melanoma) to severe neurologic deficit.

Imaging features vary with the type of primary neoplasm. On CT, metastases are typically isodense. There is usually striking perilesional edema, greater than expected for lesion size. The hypodense edema may be the only abnormality identified on noncontrast CT scan. Hyperdense metastases are seen with hemorrhagic metastases, small round cell tumors (lymphoma), and mucinous tumors (gastrointestinal adenocarcinoma). Most metastases enhance strongly following contrast on CT, exhibiting a solid or ringlike pattern. False-negative studies occur in 11.5% of patients on CT if scanned immediately following administration of the standard contrast dose. Double-dose, delayed imaging has been shown to improve the sensitivity and specificity for detecting parenchymal metastatic disease on CT.

MRI with contrast is the most sensitive imaging modality in the detection of central nervous system metastases. Signal intensity is variable. Most nonhemorrhagic lesions are hypointense on T1-weighted images and hyperintense on T2-weighted images. In metastatic melanoma with high melanin content, lesions are typically hyperintense on T1-weighted acquisition and iso- to hypointense on T2-weighted images. This finding, however, is not common, as most melanoma either is amelanotic or has low melanin content. Most melanoma will demonstrate prolonged T1 and T2 signal characteristics unless hemorrhagic (which is common). Mucinous adenocarcinoma (typically colon) and densely cellular tumors with high nuclear/cytoplasmic ratios (such as lymphoma) may also be hypointense on T2-weighted images. Hemorrhagic metastases have complex imaging characteristics, which depend on the stage of degradation of blood products. In the late stage, a hemosiderin ring may be present.

Typically, a significant amount of perilesional edema is associated with metastases relative to lesion size. The edema pattern on PD, T2, and FLAIR images follows the white matter tracts with sparing of the overlying cortex due to changes in vascular permeability (vasogenic edema pattern). Edema does not typically cross the corpus callosum or involve the cortex, which helps differentiate metastases from primary brain tumor. Cortical metastases do occur. They typically elicit very little perilesional edema, probably because of very little surrounding interstitium.

The vast majority of lesions enhance following contrast in a solid, rim, or nodular pattern. High-dose contrast (0.3 mmol/kg) has been shown to be even more sensitive in the detection of CNS metastases, particularly in the evaluation of small lesions, additional lesions, and early disease.

The differential diagnosis for multiple parenchymal enhancing lesions in the brain includes metastases, vasculitis, embolic infarcts, demyelinating disease, abscesses, multifocal glioma, and radiation necrosis. For a solitary enhancing supratentorial lesion, glioblastoma multiforme, abscess and metastases are the primary diagnostic considerations. In the posterior fossa, a solitary lesion could be metastases, hemangioblastoma, or lymphoma.

SUGGESTED READINGS

Atlas SW, Grossman RI, Gomori JM, et al. MR imaging of intracranial metastatic melanoma. *JCAT* 1987;11:577–582.

Atlas SW, Lavi E. Intra-axial brain tumors. In: Atlas SW, ed. *Magnetic resonance imaging of the brain and spine*, 2nd ed. Philadelphia: Lippincott-Raven, 1996:407–415.

Davis PC, Hudgins PA, Peterman SB, Hoffman JC Jr. Diagnosis of cerebral metastases: double-dose delayed CT vs. contrast-enhanced MR imaging. *AJNR* 1991;12:293–300.

Destian S, Sze G, Krol G, et al. MR imaging of hemorrhagic intracranial neoplasms. *AJR* 1989;152:137–144.

Egelhoff JC, Ross JS, Modic MT, et al. MR imaging of metastatic GI adenocarcinoma in brain. *AJNR* 1992;13:1221–1224.

Haustein J, Laniado M, Neindorf H-P, et al. Triple-dose versus standard-dose gadopentetate dimeglumine: a randomized study in 199 patients. *Radiology* 1993;186:855–860.

Isiklar I, Leeds NE, Fuller GN, et al. Intracranial metastatic melanoma: correlation between MR imaging characteristics and melanin content. *AJR* 1995;165:1503–1512.

Osborn AG. Miscellaneous tumors, cysts, and metastases. In: *Diagnostic neuroradiology*. St. Louis: Mosby, 1994:660–665.

Runge VM, Wells JD, Williams NM. MR imaging of an experimental model of intracranial metastatic disease: a study of lesion detection. *Invest Radiol* 1994;29:1050–1056.

Yuh WTC, Engelken JD, Muhonen MG, et al. Experience with high-dose gadolinium MR imaging in the evaluation of brain metastases. *AJNR* 1992;13:335–345.

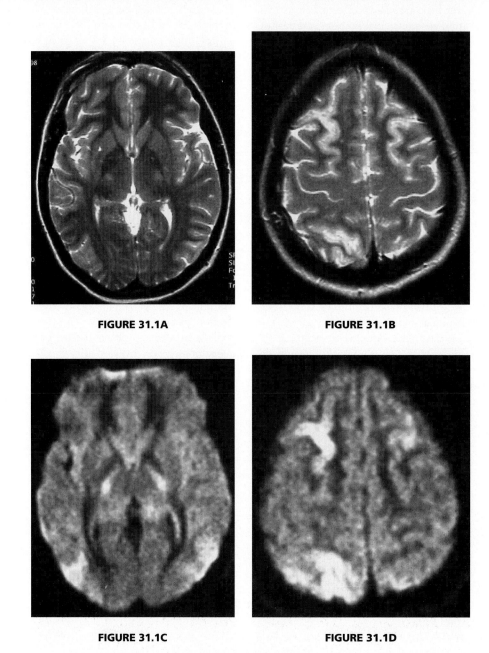

FIGURE 31.1A

FIGURE 31.1B

FIGURE 31.1C

FIGURE 31.1D

CLINICAL HISTORY

A 22-year-old female found at home obtunded.

FINDINGS

Axial T2-weighted images (Fig. 31.1A,B) demonstrate subtle hyperintense foci within the thalami bilaterally. Additionally, there is subtle gyriform high signal within the cortex along the high convexity involving the frontal and parietal lobes bilaterally in a watershed distribution. Axial diffusion-weighted images (Fig. 31.1C,D) show corresponding high-signal lesions.

DIAGNOSIS

Anoxia due to carbon monoxide poisoning.

DISCUSSION

Carbon monoxide attaches preferentially to the hemoglobin molecule, displacing oxygen. Therefore hypoxia is the mechanism of cerebral insult in carbon monoxide poisoning. The same pathophysiology applies as with asphyxia, global circulatory arrest, or any other cause of hypoxia. (See the discussion of hypoxic ischemia encephalopathy, Vol. 1, Case 55.)

SUGGESTED READINGS

Chang KH, Han MH, Kim HS, et al. Delayed encephalopathy after acute carbon monoxide intoxication: MR imaging features and distribution of cerebral white matter lesions. *Radiology* 1992;184:117–122.

Horowitz AL, Kaplan R, Sarpel G. Carbon monoxide toxicity: MR imaging in the brain. *Radiology* 1987;162:787–788.

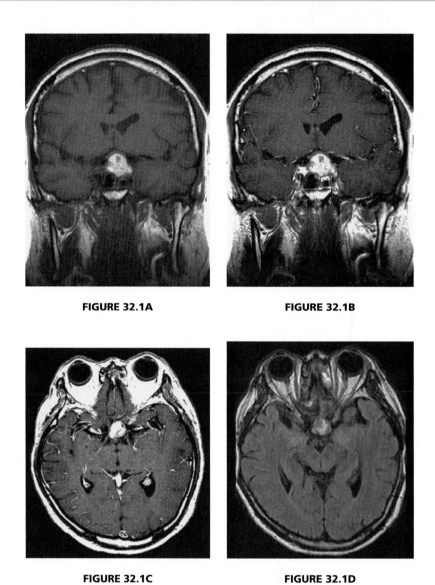

FIGURE 32.1A

FIGURE 32.1B

FIGURE 32.1C

FIGURE 32.1D

CLINICAL HISTORY

A 25-year-old female with recent-onset headache and bitemporal hemianopsia.

FINDINGS

A 2-cm mass in the pituitary fossa with suprasellar extension is causing compression of the optic chiasm. The mass has heterogeneous signal, predominantly hyperintense on unenhanced T1-weighted images (Fig. 32.1A), with heterogeneous enhancement (Fig. 32.1B,C) and mixed signal on FLAIR images (Fig. 32.1D).

DIAGNOSIS

Hemorrhagic pituitary adenoma.

DISCUSSION

Pituitary adenomas are the most common intracranial tumors to develop intratumoral hemorrhage. Hemorrhagic pituitary tumors are usually macroadenomas (40% to 80%) rather than microadenomas. The majority are prolactinomas and nonfunctioning macroadenomas. The main clinical presentation includes headache, visual field defects, and neuroendocrine symptoms. Pituitary "apoplexy" rarely occurs.

The etiology of the hemorrhage is not well understood. Several hypotheses have been suggested, including outgrowth of blood supply, impaction of the pituitary adenoma against the diaphragma sellae, and increased intracapsular pressure due to tumor growth, leading to infarction and hemorrhage. Although the association between bromocriptine and hemorrhage is well documented, the underlying mechanism is still not well established.

Submitted by Peter Brotchie, MBBS, PhD; Sattam Lingawi, MB, ChB, FRCPC; William G. Bradley, MD, PhD, FACR (Senior Editor), Long Beach Memorial Medical Center, Long Beach, CA.

SUGGESTED READING

Poussaint TY, Barnes PD, Anthony DC, et al. Hemorrhagic pituitary adenoma of adolescence. *AJNR* 1996;17:1907–1912.

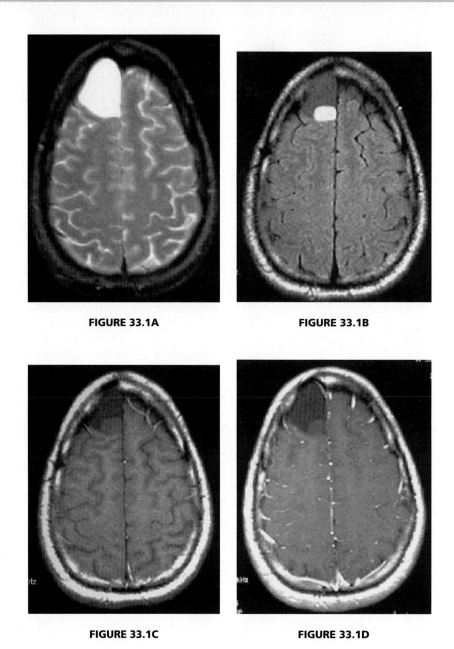

FIGURE 33.1A　　　　　　**FIGURE 33.1B**

FIGURE 33.1C　　　　　　**FIGURE 33.1D**

CLINICAL HISTORY

A 46-year-old male with headaches.

FINDINGS

T1- and T2-weighted images demonstrate a cystic extraaxial lesion in the right frontal region with signal intensity similar to that of cerebrospinal fluid (CSF) (Fig. 33.1A,C,D). In the dependent part of the lesion there is slightly increased signal intensity on the T1-weighted images and high signal intensity on FLAIR, consistent with increased protein content (Fig. 33.1B–D).

DIAGNOSIS

Hemorrhagic arachnoid cyst.

DISCUSSION

Hemorrhage into an arachnoid cyst is a rare complication. It may turn this usually asymptomatic entity into a symptomatic one. There appears to be no direct relationship between the location or size of the arachnoid cyst and the occurrence of hemorrhage. It may occur spontaneously or following trauma. Rupture of the cyst wall and bridging vessels causes bleeding into the cyst as well as the adjacent subdural space. With time the intracystic blood will form a clot that may or may not be adherent to the cyst wall. Rarely, infection and calcification of the cyst wall may also occur.

Submitted by Peter Brotchie, MBBS, PhD; Sattam Lingawi, MB, ChB, FRCPC; William G. Bradley, MD, PhD, FACR (Senior Editor), Long Beach Memorial Medical Center, Long Beach, CA.

SUGGESTED READING

Eustace S, Toland J, Stack J. CT and MRI of arachnoid cyst with complicating intracystic and subdural hemorrhage. *JCAT* 1992;16:995–997.

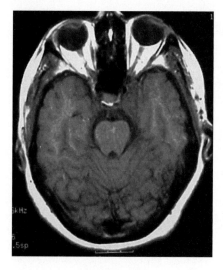

FIGURE 34.1A

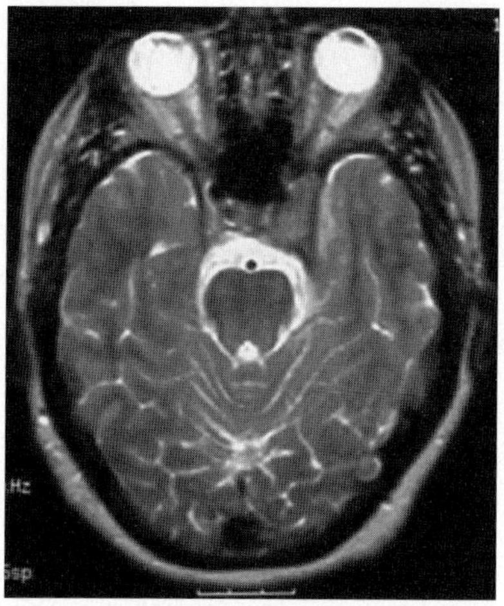

FIGURE 34.1B

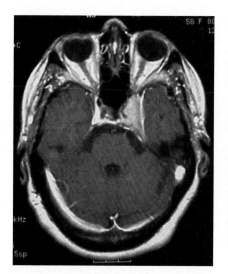

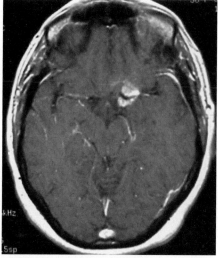

FIGURE 34.1C

FIGURE 34.1D

CLINICAL HISTORY

Left ptosis.

FINDINGS

Axial T1- and T2-weighted images (Fig. 34A,B) show a mass within the left cavernous sinus. Note convex lateral wall of the involved sinus. Following intravenous contrast (Fig. 34C,D) there is intense, homogeneous enhancement of the mass. Note extension of enhancing tumor into the left suprasellar cistern with encasement of the left middle cerebral artery. The cavernous left internal carotid artery is displaced medially.

DIAGNOSIS

Left cavernous sinus meningioma.

DISCUSSION

The specific imaging features of meningioma have been discussed elsewhere in this series. (See Vol. I, Case 76 and Vol. II, Case 21.)

A unilateral cavernous sinus mass lesion has an extensive differential diagnosis, including meningioma, schwannoma, metastasis (hematogenous or perineural), aneurysm, and carotid-cavernous fistula. Chordoma and lymphoma are less common considerations. Rarely, lipoma, epidermoid, cavernous hemangioma, and osteocartilagenous tumors can involve the cavernous sinus. Bilateral cavernous sinus abnormality can be seen with invasive pituitary adenoma, meningioma, metastases, lymphoma, and cavernous sinus thrombosis. Inflammatory pseudotumor (Talosa Hunt) and sarcoidosis can also present as a cavernous sinus mass.

Differentiating meningioma from other cavernous sinus mass lesions is difficult based on imaging features alone. Encasement of the cavernous internal carotid artery is commonly seen with cavernous sinus meningioma. There is often constriction of the involved vessel lumen, a rare finding in other tumors.

SUGGESTED READINGS

Brodac GB, Riva A, Schorner W, et al. Cavernous sinus meningiomas: an MRI study. *Neuroradiology* 1987;29:578–581.

Kucharczyk W, Montanera WJ, Becker LE. The sella turcica and parasellar region. In: Atlas SW, ed. *Magnetic resonance imaging of the brain and spine*, 2nd ed. Philadelphia: Lippincott-Raven, 1996.

Lanzino G, Hirsch NL, Pomonis S, et al. Cavernous sinus tumors: neuroradiological and neurosurgical considerations on 150 operated cases. *J Neurosurg Sci* 1992;36:183–196.

Shaffrey ME, Dolenc VV, Lanzino G, et al. Invasion of the internal carotid artery by cavernous sinus meningiomas. *Surg Neurol* 1999;52:167–171.

Zee CS, Chin T, Segall HD, et al. MR imaging of meningiomas. *Semin Ultrasound CT MR* 1992;13:154–169.

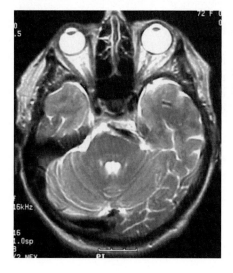 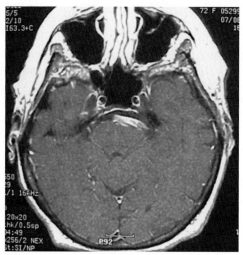

FIGURE 35.1A   **FIGURE 35.1B**

CLINICAL HISTORY

A 72-year-old female with left facial pain.

FINDINGS

Axial fast spin-echo T2-weighted and postcontrast T1-weighted image (Fig. 35.1A,B) demonstrate marked tortuosity of the basilar artery with compression of the left ventral aspect of the brainstem at the level of the dorsal root exit zone of the fifth cranial nerve. (Courtesy of Christine Colton, MD, Rush-Presbyterian-St. Luke's Medical Center, Chicago, Illinois.)

DIAGNOSIS

Basilar artery ectasia.

DISCUSSION

Dolichoectasia of the vertebrobasilar arteries with compression of the brainstem at the nerve root exit zone of the fifth and/or seventh cranial nerves is a common cause of trigeminal neuralgia and hemifacial spasm. Other etiologies include extraaxial mass lesions in the cerebellopontine angle (i.e., meningioma, acoustic schwannoma) and intraparenchymal brainstem lesions (i.e., multiple sclerosis).

The anterior inferior cerebellar artery is the most commonly implicated vessel, followed by the vertebral artery, the posterior inferior cerebellar artery, and the basilar artery in decreasing order of frequency. Increased signal within the vessel may be seen due to turbulent or slow flow. Although the ectatic vessel can be identified on MRA, the diagnosis cannot be made using MRA alone as the relationship of the ectatic vessel to the underlying parenchyma cannot be evaluated. A technique known as MR tomographic angiography has been shown to be more sensitive and specific in the diagnosis of vascular compression syndrome. This technique uses a conventional three-dimensional time-of-flight MRA with reformatted submillimeter images in the coronal, sagittal, and oblique plane. The window and level are adjusted to allow visualization of both the vascular structures and adjacent brainstem parenchyma as well as the nerve root exit zones.

Studies have shown asymptomatic control subjects with neurovascular compression in up to 20% of cases. Although neurovascular compression may be asymptomatic, in the setting of hemifacial spasm, the demonstration of vascular compression at the seventh nerve root exit zone on MRI implicates neurovascular compression as the cause of the symptoms.

SUGGESTED READINGS

Bernardi B, Zimmerman RA, Savino PJ, et al. Magnetic resonance tomographic angiography in the investigation of hemifacial spasm. *Neuroradiology* 1993;35:606–611.

Felber S, Birbamer G, Aichner F, et al. Magnetic resonance imaging and angiography in hemifacial spasm. *Neuroradiology* 1992;34:413–416.

Furuya Y, Ryu H, Uemura K, et al. MRI of intracranial neurovascular compression. *JCAT* 1992;16:503–505.

Ho SL, Cheng PW, Wong WC, et al. A case-controlled MRI/MRA study of neurovascular contact in hemifacial spasm. *Neurology* 1999;53:2132–2139.

Tash R, DeMerritt J, Sze G, et al. Hemifacial spasm: MR imaging features. *AJNR* 1991;12:839–842.

Tien RD, Wilkins RH. MRA delineation of the vertebral-basilar system in patients with hemifacial spasm and trigeminal neuralgia. *AJNR* 1993;14:34–36.

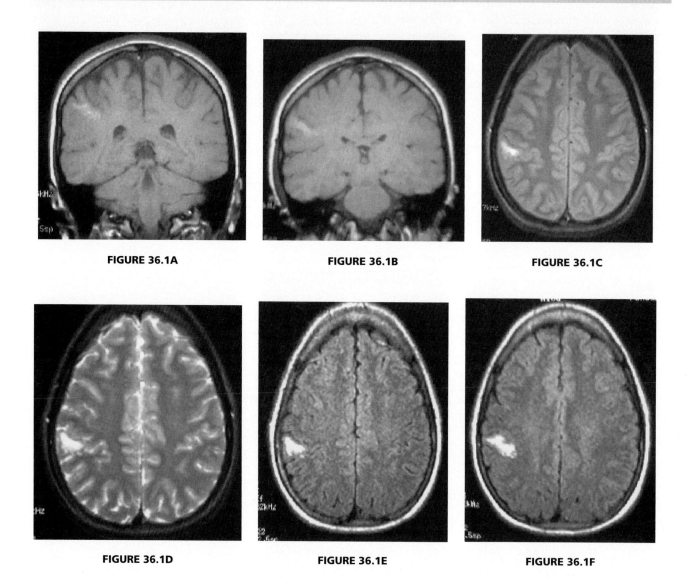

FIGURE 36.1A FIGURE 36.1B FIGURE 36.1C

FIGURE 36.1D FIGURE 36.1E FIGURE 36.1F

CLINICAL HISTORY

A 20-year-old female with a history of chronic epilepsy.

FINDINGS

A lesion is present within the right central sulcus, extending to the cortical surface (Fig. 36.1A–F). The lesion is slightly hyperintense on T1-weighted imaging and hyperintense on proton-density, T2-weighted, and FLAIR images. No significant mass effect is evident.

DIAGNOSIS

Dysembryoplastic neuroectodermal tumor (DNET).

DISCUSSION

DNET was first recognized as a separate entity in 1988 and has recently been included as a mixed neurologic tumor in the World Health Organization (WHO) classification of brain tumors. They usually present in early adulthood with epilepsy and are most commonly located in the lateral aspect of the temporal lobes. Histopathologically, DNET is a benign intracortical multilocular lesion composed of glial and neuronal elements. They share several important features with gangliogliomas and glioneuronal malformations.

On MRI these lesions have low signal intensity on T1-weighted images and may or may not enhance after gadolinium administration. T2-weighted images show the lesion to be of high signal intensity. Multinodularity and multicystic appearance is rare but helps to differentiate it from other conditions associated with chronic epilepsy. Calcification is rarely present. These tumors do not cause any mass effect or edema until they reach a large size.

Modern MR techniques with high resolution and high contrast permit detection of lesions a few millimeters in size. Following mesial temporal sclerosis, benign temporal lobe tumors are the second most frequent lesions to cause chronic seizures. Therefore MRI should be routinely used to examine patients with chronic epilepsy.

Submitted by Sattam Lingawi, MB, ChB, FRCPC; Peter Brotchie, MBBS, PhD; William G. Bradley, MD, PhD, FACR (Senior Editor), Long Beach Memorial Medical Center, Long Beach, CA.

SUGGESTED READING

Ostertun BO, Wolf HK, Campos MG, et al. Dysembryoplastic neuroectodermal tumors: MR and CT evaluation. *AJNR* 1996;17:419–430.

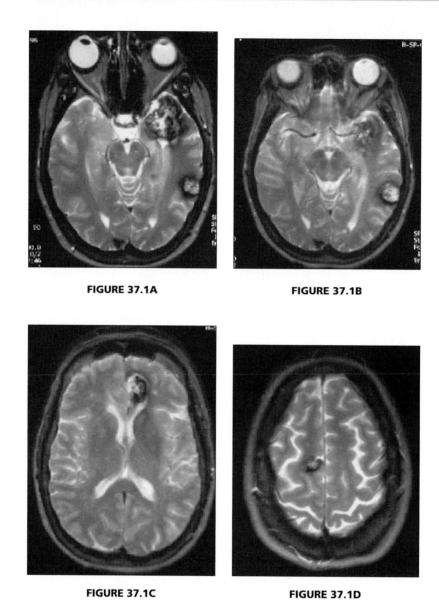

FIGURE 37.1A

FIGURE 37.1B

FIGURE 37.1C

FIGURE 37.1D

CLINICAL HISTORY

A 49-year-old female with headaches.

FINDINGS

There are multiple lesions of variable size and signal intensity with low-intensity rims (Fig. 37.1A-D). The largest lesion is in the left anterior temporal lobe (Fig. 37.1A,B). Smaller lesions are seen more posteriorly. Other lesions are identified in the left parasagittal anterior frontal lobe (Fig. 37.1C) and the right frontal lobe (Fig. 37.1D).

DIAGNOSIS

Multiple cavernous hemangiomas.

DISCUSSION

There are four basic types of intracranial vascular malformations: cavernous angiomas, venous angiomas, capillary telangiectasias, and arteriovenous malformations. Cavernous hemangiomas are the most commonly identified vascular malformation on MRI. They are seen in both sexes and in all age groups (mean age of presentation = 30 years). Multiplicity is identified in approximately 50% of sporadic and 80% of familial cases. These lesions are often asymptomatic; however, they have an inherent tendency to bleed that results in variable clinical presentations, depending on the anatomic location. The most common symptoms are headache and seizures.

On MRI these lesions are often described as "popcorn" or "mulberry" lesions because of their mixed core signal intensity that represents variable stages of hemorrhage. A dark hemosiderin rim causes a negative blooming effect on T2-weighted spin-echo conventional images (although this is less pronounced on fast spin-echo images). T2-weighted gradient echo sequences are the most sensitive for detection of hemosiderin due to the accentuation of the magnetic susceptibility effect; hence they are useful for detecting these conditions.

The differential diagnosis includes other vascular malformations, hemorrhagic metastases, and thrombosed arteriovenous malformations.

Submitted by Peter Brotchie, MBBS, PhD; Sattam Lingawi, MB, ChB, FRCPC; William G. Bradley, MD, PhD, FACR (Senior Editor), Long Beach Memorial Medical Center, Long Beach, CA.

SUGGESTED READINGS

Rigamonti D, Hadley MN, Drayer BP, et al. Cerebral cavernous malformations: incidence and familial occurrence. *N Engl J Med* 1988;319:343–347.

Tomlinson FH. Angiographically occult vascular malformations. *Neurosurgery* 1994;34:792–799.

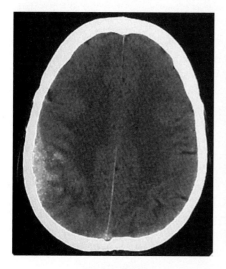

FIGURE 38.1A

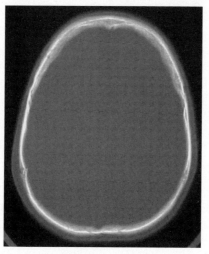

FIGURE 38.1B

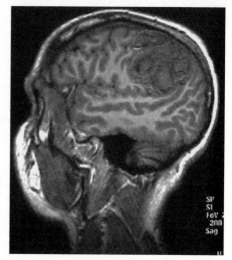

FIGURE 38.1C

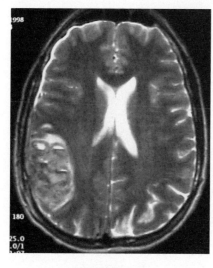

FIGURE 38.1D

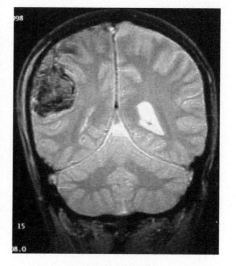

FIGURE 38.1E

CLINICAL HISTORY

A 41-year-old male with head trauma.

FINDINGS

Axial noncontrast CT scan (Fig. 38.1A) demonstrates multifocal regions of high density within the cortex and subcortical white matter of the right parietal lobe. Additionally, there is an apparent extraaxial collection of high-density material along the inner table in the same location. Bone windows (Fig. 38.1B) demonstrate a nondisplaced fracture of the right parietal bone overlying the hematoma. There is hypointense signal in the same distribution on the sagittal T1-weighted acquisition (Fig. 38.1C). Axial T2-weighted images (Fig. 38.1D) show a large isointense mass within the right parietal lobe with several high-signal fluid levels. Additionally, there is perifocal high signal consistent with edema. The extraaxial collection is intermediate in signal. Coronal gradient-echo acquisition (Fig. 38.1E) demonstrates very low signal within the mass consistent with blood products. Note the effacement of the adjacent cortical sulci as well as mild effacement of the right lateral ventricle.

DIAGNOSIS

Right parietal fracture with underlying epidural and parenchymal hematoma.

DISCUSSION

Epidural hematoma contains a higher percentage of oxygenated blood than most subdural hematomas, as frequently the bleed has an arterial (as opposed to venous) component. Also, rebleeding is seen adding fresh blood product with greater oxygen content. Therefore lower signal intensity may be seen on T1-weighted images as opposed to the high signal provided by methemoglobin in the more subsequent stages of hemoglobin degradation. Gradient-echo sequences are quite sensitive to deoxyhemoglobin, thus will show low signal within even fresh blood collections. Blood-fluid levels are more readily demonstrated on MR than on CT images, due to the differential signal provided by the deoxyhemoglobin-laden red cells that are dependent within such hematomas and yielding low signal, as compared with the supernatant serum that shows high signal on T2-weighted images. The role of MR in acute head trauma is typically secondary to CT, but MR will frequently show a greater extent of brain disease than that depicted with CT.

SUGGESTED READINGS

Atlas SW, Mark AS, Grossman RI, et al. Intracranial hemorrhage: gradient-echo MR imaging at 1.5 T. *Radiology* 1988;168:803–807.
Hayman LA, Pagani JJ, Kirkpatrick JB, et al. Pathophysiology of acute intracerebral and subarachnoid hemorrhage: applications to MR imaging. *AJNR* 1989;10:457–461.

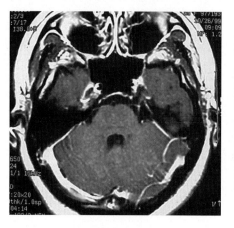 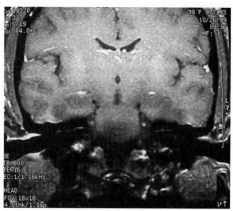

FIGURE 39.1A   **FIGURE 39.1B**

CLINICAL HISTORY

A 39-year-old female with trigeminal neuralgia.

FINDINGS

Axial and coronal postcontrast T1-weighted acquisitions (Fig. 39.1A,B) demonstrate abnormal enhancement of the cisternal portion of the left fifth cranial nerve. No abnormal enhancing lesion is seen within the brainstem or Meckel's cave. There is no focal enlargement of the trigeminal nerve.

DIAGNOSIS

Nonspecific trigeminal neuritis.

DISCUSSION

Enhancement of the trigeminal nerve can be seen with nonspecific trigeminal neuralgia (or any other neuritis, including tic douloureux). Differentiation from neuroma, carcinomatous perineural spread, or sarcoid can only be made on the basis of morphologic examination and evolution. (The latter conditions produce persistent enlargement of the nerve, as opposed to the disappearance of enhancement on 6 to 12 week follow up studies with neuritis.) Acute disseminated encephalomyelitis can produce a picture indistinguishable from neuritis but is usually associated with multifocal involvement and the history of previous vaccination or viral syndrome.

SUGGESTED READINGS

Majoie CB, Hulsmans FJ, Casteligns JA, et al. Symptoms and signs related to the trigeminal nerve: diagnostic yield of MR imaging. *Radiology* 1998;209:557–562.

Savas A, Deda H, Erden E, et al. Differential diagnosis of idiopathic inflammatory trigeminal sensory neuropathy from neuroma with a biopsy: case report. *Neurosurgery* 1999;45:1246–1250.

Yang J, Simonson TM, Ruprecht A, et al. Magnetic resonance imaging used to assess patients with trigeminal neuralgia. *Oral Surg Oral Med Oral Pathol Oral Radiol Endod* 1996;81:343–350.

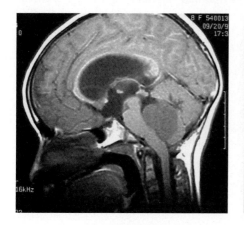

FIGURE 40.1A

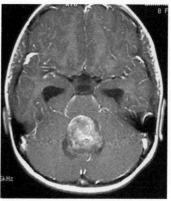

FIGURE 40.1B

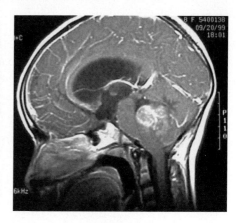

FIGURE 40.1C

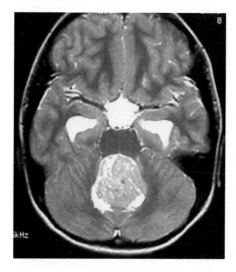

FIGURE 40.1D

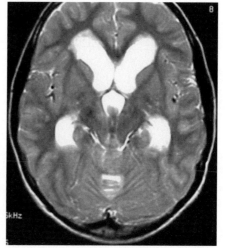

FIGURE 40.1E

CLINICAL HISTORY

An 8-year-old female with headaches and ataxia.

FINDINGS

Sagittal precontrast and axial and sagittal postcontrast T1-weighted images (Fig. 40.1A–C) demonstrate a large heterogeneously enhancing intermediate-signal mass within the posterior fossa. The mass is round in contour and appears to arise from the roof of the fourth ventricle. The mass expands the fourth ventricle and appears separate from the brainstem. There is mass effect along the dorsal aspect of the pons and medulla. There is obstructive hy-drocephalus. There is downward displacement of the cerebellar tonsils. Note intermediate signal intensity on the T2-weighted acquisition. There is abnormal high signal surrounding the frontal horns of the lateral ventricles (Fig. 40.1D,E) due to transependymal flow of cerebrospinal fluid. (Courtesy of Cornel Overbeek, MD, Rush-Presbyterian-St. Luke's Medical Center, Chicago, Illinois.)

DIAGNOSIS

Medulloblastoma.

DISCUSSION

Medulloblastoma is the most common childhood tumor to occur in the posterior fossa and is the prototype of the broad spectrum of tumors known as primitive neuroectodermal tumor (PNET). It accounts for 15% to 25% of all pediatric brain tumors. Medulloblastoma is much less common in the adult population and accounts for only 1% of brain tumors. The average age at diagnosis is 7 years.

About 80% of pediatric medulloblastomas occur in the midline (whereas adult medulloblastomas are more often lateral and hemispheric). The site of origin is the middle and inferior aspect of the anterior cerebellar vermis. Histologically, medulloblastomas are dense, hypercellular tumors primarily composed of small cells with scant cytoplasm. It is the dense cellularity and high nuclear/cytoplasmic ratio that presumably accounts for their intermediate to low signal on T2-weighted acquisition. On CT, the tumors are solid, well-defined, iso- to hyperdense masses. Regions of cystic change, hemorrhage, and necrosis are uncommon. Approximately 20% have foci of calcification; 90% enhance. Cerebrospinal fluid spread and solid central nervous system metastasis are common (40%). Interestingly, metastasis and recurrent tumor may not enhance. Relapse is common (40%), usually occurring within the first 2 years. The overall 10-year survival is 60%; children under 3 years of age have a poorer prognosis regarding both survival and quality of life.

Differential diagnosis of posterior fossa mass in a child includes ependymoma, astrocytoma (brainstem or cerebellar), choroid plexus tumor, and metastasis.

SUGGESTED READINGS

Koci TM, Chiang F, Mehringer CM, et al. Adult cerebellar medulloblastoma: imaging features with emphasis on MR findings. *AJNR* 1993;14:929–939.

Levy RA, Bliavas M, Muraszko K, et al. Desmoplastic medulloblastoma: MR findings. *AJNR* 1997;18:1364–1366.

Luh GY, Bird CR. Imaging of brain tumors in the pediatric population. *Neuroimaging Clin North Am* 1999;9:691–716.

Meyers SP, Kemp SS, Tarr RW. MR imaging features of medulloblastomas. *AJNR* 1992;158:859–865.

Rorke LB, Trojanowski JQ, Lee VM, et al. Primitive neuroectodermal tumors of the central nervous system. *Brain Pathol* 1997;7:765–784.

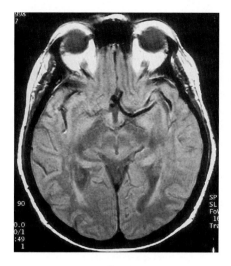

FIGURE 41.1A

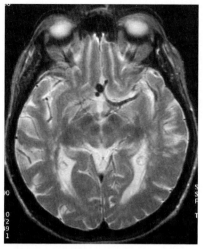

FIGURE 41.1B

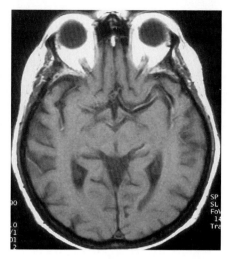

FIGURE 41.1C

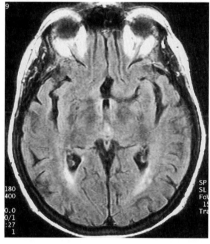

FIGURE 41.1D

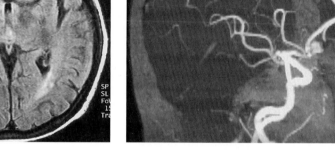

FIGURE 41.1E

CLINICAL HISTORY

A 78-year-old female complaining of headaches.

FINDINGS

There is a 7-mm low-intensity rounded mass in the intrahemispheric fissure just anterior to the circle of Willis. This is best seen on the proton-density and T2-weighted images (Fig. 41.1B,C) and is barely seen at all on the T1-weighted and FLAIR images (Fig. 41.1A,D). The lack of signal on both T1- and T2-weighted techniques is typical of rapidly flowing blood.

DIAGNOSIS

Anterior communicating artery aneurysm.

DISCUSSION

The low signal on both T1- and T2-weighted images is more typical of a "flow void" than of a magnetic susceptibility effect (which would be darker on a T2-weighted image than on a T1-weighted image). Flow voids can be due to rapidly flowing blood (as in this case) or cerebrospinal fluid (CSF) (as is frequently seen in the aqueduct in patients with communicating hydrocephalus). Other causes of signal void include dense calcification or other solids (e.g., foreign bodies or plastic prostheses) that do not contain mobile protons to give an MR signal. Air and metal can also generate signal voids; however, there tends to be a bright border (inflection zone) because of the distortion of the magnetic field. The signal loss due to metallic, paramagnetic (e.g., hemosiderin), or diamagnetic (e.g., air) susceptibility effects is more marked on a $T2^*$-weighted (low flip angle) gradient-echo image than on a conventional spin echo and is minimized on a fast spin-echo technique.

It is important to note that the aneurysm is barely seen at all on the FLAIR sequence. Although FLAIR is superb for parenchymal abnormalities abutting the CSF, it is very poor at detecting low-intensity abnormalities within the subarachnoid space. Such abnormalities are optimally seen on T2-weighted images (Fig. 41.1B) and, if recognized, should be followed with an MR angiogram (Fig. 41.1E).

Analysis of the conventional MR images and the MR angiogram demonstrates a 7-mm aneurysm angling anteriorly and to the right with a narrow neck. This information is important to the interventional neuroradiologist who may be considering an endovascular procedure or to the neurosurgeon who may be considering clipping the aneurysm.

SUGGESTED READINGS

Bradley WG. Fast spin-echo and echo-planar imaging. In: Stark DD, Bradley WG, eds. *Magnetic resonance imaging,* 3rd ed. St. Louis: Mosby, 1999:125–158.

Bradley WG. Flow phenomena. In: Stark DD, Bradley WG, eds. *Magnetic resonance imaging,* 3rd ed. St. Louis: Mosby, 1999:231–256.

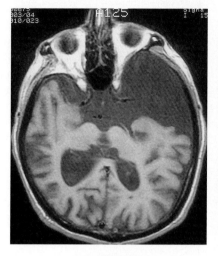

FIGURE 42.1A

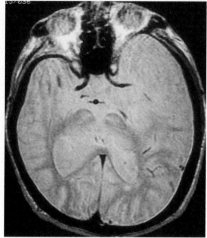

FIGURE 42.1B

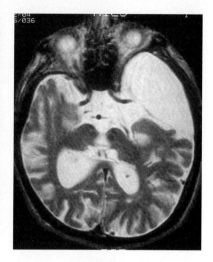

FIGURE 42.1C

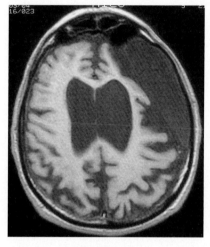

FIGURE 42.1D

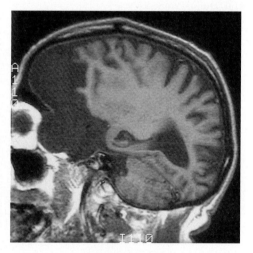

FIGURE 42.1E

CLINICAL HISTORY

A 78-year-old male with headaches.

FINDINGS

There is a very large cerebrospinal fluid (CSF) collection anterior to the left temporal lobe extending over the left frontal convexity. Although the sulci are flattened, there is no additional mass effect. The cortical vessels are applied closely to the gyri rather than floating freely in this CSF collection (Fig. 42.1A–E).

DIAGNOSIS

Arachnoid cyst.

DISCUSSION

Arachnoid cysts are congenital abnormalities that form at the same time as the developing brain. For this reason they replace brain rather than displacing it. The only evidence of mass effect is locally, where the cortical gyri are somewhat flattened. Since these cysts arise from the arachnoid membrane, they tend to push vessels in the subarachnoid space directly against the gyri. This feature helps distinguish the diagnosis of an enlarged subarachnoid space (in which the vessels could be positioned anywhere within the subarachnoid space) from arachnoid cysts (where the vessels are forced against the gyri). This latter condition can also be seen following trauma when a rent in the arachnoid results in a CSF collection in the subdural space, which also forces the vessels in the subarachnoid space against the gyri.

Uncomplicated arachnoid cysts are of CSF intensity. Those that have bled or have become infected have a higher protein content and therefore appear brighter than CSF on proton-density-weighted and FLAIR images. Arachnoid cysts can also be distinguished from epidermoid cysts in that the former are dark on diffusion imaging and the latter are bright.

Submitted by William G. Bradley, MD, PhD, FACR (Senior Editor), Long Beach Memorial Medical Center, Long Beach, CA.

SUGGESTED READING

Grollimus JM, Wilson CB, Newton TH. Paramesencephalic arachnoid cysts. *Neurology* 1976;26:128.

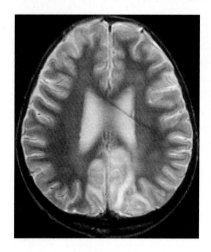

FIGURE 43.1A

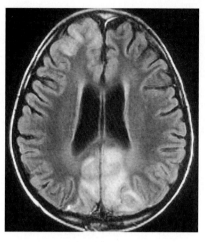

FIGURE 43.1B

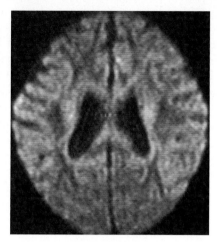

FIGURE 43.1C

CLINICAL HISTORY

An 11-year-old male on chemotherapy for acute lymphocytic leukemia (ALL) presents acutely with "stroke."

FINDINGS

Parasagittal areas of high signal are noted in the posterior frontal, parietal, occipital, and cerebellar regions on T2-weighted and FLAIR images (Fig. 43.1A,B), which are (unexpectedly) normal on the EPI diffusion images (Fig. 43.1C).

DIAGNOSIS

Hypertensive encephalopathy.

DISCUSSION

Hypertensive encephalopathy, or "posterior reversible encephalopathy syndrome," results from transudation of fluid across an otherwise intact (Fig. 43.1A,B) capillary wall, giving the appearance of vasogenic edema when, in fact, the blood-brain barrier is intact (sometimes called *reversible vasogenic edema*). Follow-up examination 30 days later demonstrate essentially normal findings without evidence of expected gliosis (had there been true infarction). This tends to be more prominent in the posterior circulation since the sympathetic enervation to the anterior circulation is greater. This pattern can be seen in patients in hypertensive crisis, transplant patients on cyclosporin, pregnant patients with eclampsia or preeclampsia, and children on intrathecal chemotherapy where relatively minor elevations in blood pressure are sufficient to produce this transudation. The key to the diagnosis is the parasagittal location and lack of positive findings on diffusion imaging when ischemia would be very bright. (For this reason we perform diffusion imaging on every MRI of the brain performed at our institution.)

Submitted by William G. Bradley, MD, PhD, FACR (Senior Editor), Long Beach Memorial Medical Center, Long Beach, CA.

SUGGESTED READING

Cooney MJ, Bradley WG, Symko SC, et al. Hypertensive encephalopathy: complication in children treated for myeloproliferative disorders: report of three cases. *Radiology* 2000;214:711–716.

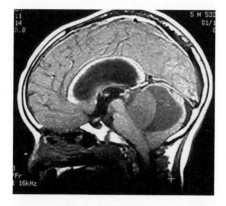

FIGURE 44.1A

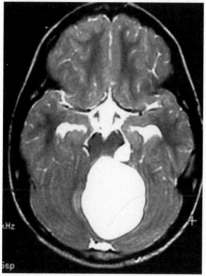

FIGURE 44.1B

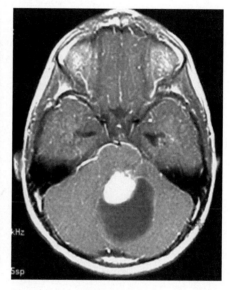

FIGURE 44.1C

CLINICAL HISTORY

A 5-year-old male with history of ataxia.

FINDINGS

Sagittal T1-weighted images (Fig. 44.1A) demonstrate a large cystic mass containing an isointense nodule within the posterior fossa. The mass effaces the fourth ventricle with secondary obstructive hydrocephalus. There is mild mass effect along the dorsal aspect of the brainstem. There is downward displacement of the cerebellar tonsils. Axial T2- and postcontrast T1-weighted images (Fig. 44.1B,C) show the nodule within high signal-cystic fluid on the T2-weighted acquisition; intense enhancement of the nodule is seen on postcontrast acquisition. There is effacement with rightward displacement of the midbrain.

DIAGNOSIS

Cystic astrocytoma.

DISCUSSION

The cerebellar astrocytoma is one of the most common posterior fossa tumors in the pediatric population. Of all posterior fossa astrocytomas, 85% are histologically pilocytic astrocytomas. These tumors represent one of the most benign forms of glial neoplasm, and boast the longest survival rate of all primary gliomas (94% at 25 years). Their peak incidence is in the first two decades of life but can present in patients up to 40 years of age. The minority of cerebellar astrocytomas (15%) are infiltrative, fibrillary-type tumors, which usually occur in an older age group. These are more commonly solid lesions, often associated with hemorrhage and necrosis. Common presenting symptoms include headache, vomiting, brainstem dysfunction, and ataxia.

The classic cerebellar pilocytic astrocytoma, seen in this case, presents as a large, well-circumscribed cyst with solid, intensely enhancing mural nodule. The mass may be midline or hemispheric. The cyst wall is typically not lined with epithelial tissue but consists of nonneoplastic compressed glial tissue that does not enhance. In this case, resection of the mural nodule alone is adequate to prevent recurrence of tumor. If the cyst wall enhances, usually indicating a solid tumor with central cystic necrosis, neoplastic cells line the cyst, and a complete resection is required. The fourth ventricle is typically effaced and displaced rather than expanded, an important finding when trying to differentiate posterior fossa neoplasms. Hydrocephalus is common at presentation. The solid portion of the tumor is isointense to normal brain on T2-weighted images. The cystic portion is usually isointense to slightly hyperintense to cerebrospinal fluid (CSF), depending on the protein content. The signal characteristics are generally more homogeneous as compared with ependymoma, although heterogeneity does not exclude the diagnosis. Approximately 20% of cerebellar astrocytomas calcify. In classic pilocytic astrocytoma, hemorrhage is rare and there is notable absence of perifocal edema.

SUGGESTED READINGS

Atlas SW, Lavi E. Intra-axial brain tumors. In: Atlas SW, ed. *Magnetic resonance imaging of the brain and spine*, 2nd ed. Philadelphia: Lippincott-Raven, 1996:353,371.

Campbell JW, Pollack IF. Cerebellar astrocytomas in children. *J Neurooncol* 1996;28:223–231.

Gjerris F, Kinken L. Long-term prognosis in children with benign cerebellar astrocytomas. *J Neurosurg* 1978;49:179.

Lee Y-Y, Van Tassel P, Burner JM, et al. Juvenile pilocytic astrocytomas: CT and MR characteristics. *AJNR* 1989;10:363–370.

Russell DS, Rubinstein LF. *Pathology of tumors of the nervous system,* 5th ed. Baltimore: Williams & Wilkins, 1989.

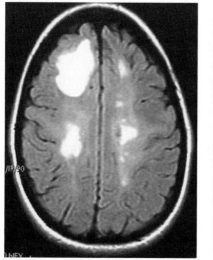

FIGURE 45.1A

FIGURE 45.1B

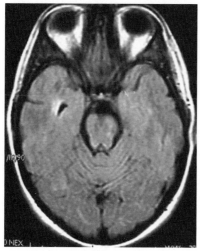

FIGURE 45.1C

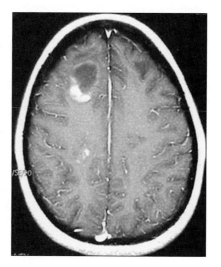

FIGURE 45.1D

CLINICAL HISTORY

A 30-year-old female with leg and arm weakness.

FINDINGS

Axial FLAIR images (Fig. 45.1A,B) demonstrate small linear foci of high signal within the deep periventricular white matter. The long axis of these lesions lay perpendicular to the axis of the lateral ventricles. Additionally, there are larger amorphous regions of high signal within the centrum semiovale bilaterally. There are smaller lesions within the left dorsolateral aspect of the pons and the deep white matter adjacent to the right temporal horn (Fig. 45.1C). Following intravenous contrast (Fig. 45.1D), there is enhancement of multiple tiny periventricular lesions as well as peripheral enhancement of the large lesion within the right frontal lobe (a "target" lesion). (Courtesy of Srilatha Kannam, MD, Rush-Presbyterian-St. Luke's Medical Center, Chicago, Illinois.)

DIAGNOSIS

Tumefactive multiple sclerosis.

DISCUSSION

The cause of multiple sclerosis (MS) is uncertain, but MS may be due to an autoimmune-mediated demyelination in genetically susceptible individuals. Symptom onset is usually between the ages of 20 and 40, with a female predominance, especially when it occurs in children and adolescents. MS patients usually present with multifocal neurologic deficits. The clinical course is one of prolonged relapsing/remitting disease. Disease can shift into a chronic-progressive phase and, rarely, a fulminant type (MS of Marburg type), which is associated with a rapid clinical decline with substantial morbidity and mortality.

Pathologically, MS "plaques" appear as edematous white matter lesions. Necrosis and atrophy with cystic change are common in chronic lesions. Hemorrhage and calcification are rare. Microscopically, one sees destruction of myelin and myelin-producing oligodendrocytes with relative sparing of the axon.

The classic imaging feature is multiple ovoid periventricular lesions that are oriented perpendicularly to the long axis of the lateral ventricles (seen in 85% of MS patients). This pattern of disease correlates with the propensity of the demyelinating process to occur around subependymal and deep white matter medullary veins. These fingerlike perivascular lesions emanating from the ventricular margin are commonly referred to as *Dawson's fingers*. The next most common location for MS plaques is the corpus callosum, typically at the callososeptal interface. These lesions are most commonly found along the inferior surface of the corpus callosum and are best seen on sagittal PD, T2-weighted, or FLAIR images. Involvement of the internal capsule, pons, periaqueductal gray matter, floor of the fourth ventricle, and brachium pontis is common. MS plaques can involve the cortex. MS plaques are typically multifocal; however, a large solitary plaque can occur. Infratentorial lesions (brainstem and cerebellum) are uncommon in adult disease but are frequently seen in children and adolescents with MS.

CT scans are often normal in early MS; therefore MRI is the imaging modality of choice. When present, MS lesions appear iso- to hypodense on CT with variable enhancement. On MRI, MS plaques are iso- to hypointense on T1-weighted images and hyperintense on T2-weighted and FLAIR acquisition. FLAIR images are particularly helpful in lesion identification because of the suppression of cerebrospinal fluid (CSF) signal within subjacent ventricles, making periventricular MS lesions more conspicuous. Because there are several causes for multiple high-signal periventricular lesions in the brain, some criteria have been established for the MR diagnosis of MS. These include three or more discrete lesions that measure 5 mm or greater, a periventricular or callososeptal distribution, and a compatible clinical history. Identification of the typical oblong periventricular lesions (Dawson's finger appearance) is also suggestive of the diagnosis. MS lesions can appear as a lesion within a lesion or as a target lesion on T1-weighted and PD images. This imaging appearance is thought to represent a central demyelinating plaque with perifocal edema (which creates the outer lesion or halo) or possibly varying degrees of demyelination within a single lesion. In severe disease the discrete periventricular lesions can become confluent. In approximately 10% of patients with long-standing MS, abnormal hypointense basal ganglia related to iron deposition have been described. Most MS plaques do not enhance following contrast. Enhancement is typically transient and is thought to occur during the active phase of demyelination. Enhancement can be solid or ringlike. A large, solitary enhancing MS plaque can be indistinguishable from tumor or abscess. The large MS plaques are referred to as *tumefactive* MS (as seen in this case).

Plaques of Balo concentric sclerosis exhibit a unique imaging pattern of concentric rings surrounding an acute MS plaque. They are thought to represent free radicals within the macrophage layer at the margin of an acute demyelinating lesion. The rings are typically multiple and slightly hyperintense on T1-weighted images.

Although MRI is extremely sensitive in the detection of MS plaques, the extent of disease seen on conventional MRI does not correlate well with the clinical status of the patient with regard to disability. Notwithstanding the relative correlation between "active" disease and contrast enhancement on conventional MRI, there is a lack of specificity in the ability to determine the precise biochemical nature of MS lesions using conventional MRI. In this regard, proton MR spectroscopy and magnetization transfer MR techniques are now being studied and used to better characterize the "activity" of MS lesions to monitor treatment response and predict clinical outcome.

SUGGESTED READINGS

Edwards-Brown MK, Bonnin JM. White matter diseases. In: Atlas SW, ed. *Magnetic resonance imaging of the brain and spine*, 2nd ed. Philadelphia: Lippincott-Raven, 1996:653–674.

Filippi M. Magnetization transfer imaging to monitor the evolution of individual MS lesions. *Neurology* 1999;53[Suppl 3]:S18–S22.

Gean-Marton AD, Vezina LG, Marton KI, et al. Abnormal corpus callosum: a sensitive and specific indicator of multiple sclerosis. *Radiology* 1991;180:215–221.

Giang DW, Podure KR, Eskin TA, et al. Multiple sclerosis masquerading as a mass lesion. *Neuroradiology* 1992;34:150–154.

Grossman RI, Lenkinski RE, Ramer KN, et al. MR proton spectroscopy in multiple sclerosis. *AJNR* 1992;13:1535–1543.

Horowitz AL, Kaplan RD, Grewe G, et al. The ovoid lesions: a new MR observation in patients with multiple sclerosis. *AJNR* 1989;10:303–305.

Nesbit GM, Forbes GS, Scheithauer BW, et al. Multiple sclerosis: histopathologic and MR and/or CT correlation in 37 cases at biopsy and three cases at autopsy. *Radiology* 1991;180:467–474.

Offenbacher H, Fazekas F, Schmidt R, et al. Assessment of MRI criteria for a diagnosis of MS. *Neurology* 1993;43:905–909.

Osborn AG, Harnsberger HR, Smoker WRK, et al. Multiple sclerosis in adolescents: CT and MR findings. *AJNR* 1990;11:489–494.

Powell T, Sussman JG, Davies-Jones GAB. MR imaging in acute multiple sclerosis: ring-like appearance in plaques suggesting the presence of paramagnetic free radicals. *AJNR* 1992;13:1544–1546.

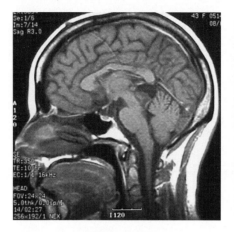

FIGURE 46.1A   FIGURE 46.1B

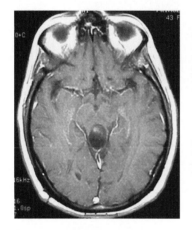
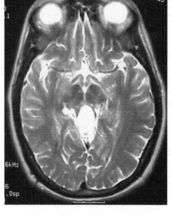
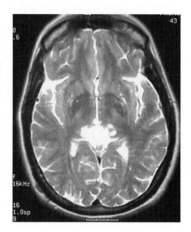

FIGURE 46.1C   FIGURE 46.1D   FIGURE 46.1E

CLINICAL HISTORY

Diplopia with vertical gaze.

FINDINGS

Sagittal noncontrast T1-weighted acquisition (Fig. 46.1A) demonstrates a heterogeneous mass in the region of the tectal plate with associated cyst formation. Pre- and postcontrast axial T1-weighted images (Fig. 46.1B,C) demonstrate subtle enhancement of the nodular portion of the mass. Axial T2-weighted images (Fig. 46.1D,E) show a well-defined hyperintense cystic lesion along the dorsal aspect of the midbrain with intermediate signal in the region of the nodular component. There is extension of signal abnormality into the thalami bilaterally.

DIAGNOSIS

Tectal glioma.

DISCUSSION

Half of all primary brain tumors are of glial cell origin and more than 75% of gliomas are astrocytomas. Other glial cell tumors include oligodendroglioma, ependymoma, and choroid plexus papilloma/carcinoma.

Most tectal plate gliomas (as seen in this case) are low-grade astrocytomas. Low-grade tumors usually occur in children and young adults (20 to 40 years of age). A tectal plate glioma typically presents with signs of increased intracranial pressure related to obstructive hydrocephalus at the level of the Sylvian aqueduct. Diplopia is a common focal finding.

Tectal gliomas are slow-growing tumors, which are often treated with ventriculoperitoneal shunt alone. Long-term survival (years after initial diagnosis) is common. Chemotherapy and radiation are used in progressive lesions.

At imaging, there is enlargement and distortion of the tectum with hyperintense signal on T2-weighted images. The T1-weighted signal and enhancement characteristics are variable. Cystic change and calcification can be present. Perifocal edema, hemorrhage, and enhancement are uncommon.

SUGGESTED READINGS

Bognar L, Turjman F, Villany E. Tectal plate gliomas: Part II. CT scan and MR imaging of the tectal gliomas. *Acta Neurochir (Wien)* 1994;127:48–54.

Boydston WR, Sanford RA, Muhlbauer MS, et al. Gliomas of the tectum and periaqueductal region of the mesencephalon. *Pediatr Neurosurg* 1991–92;17:234–238.

Squeres LA, Allen JC, Abbott R, et al. Focal tectal tumors: management and prognosis. *Neurology* 1994;44:953–956.

Vandertop WP, Hoffman HJ, Drake JM. Focal midbrain tumors in childhood. *Neurosurgery* 1992;31:186–194.

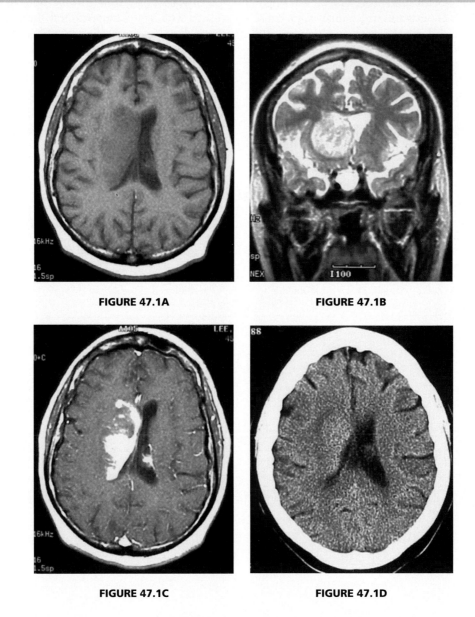

FIGURE 47.1A

FIGURE 47.1B

FIGURE 47.1C

FIGURE 47.1D

CLINICAL HISTORY

A 45-year-old female with history of systemic lupus erythematosus on long-term steroids.
The patient has altered mental status with intermittent lethargy and bizarre behavior.

FINDINGS

Axial T1-weighted and coronal fast spin-echo T2-weighted images (Fig. 47.1A,B) demonstrate a large homogeneous mass centered within the right basal ganglia. There is associated mass effect with effacement of the right lateral ventricle as well as mild shift of the midline structures toward the left. The mass is intermediate in signal on T1-weighted acquisition and intermediate to slightly hyperintense on the T2-weighted images. Following intervenous contrast (Fig.

47.1C), there is intense heterogeneous enhancement of the mass as well as enhancement along the ependymal surface of the right lateral ventricle. There is a smaller focus of enhancement within the posterior body of the left lateral ventricle.

Axial noncontrast CT demonstrates a high-density mass (Fig. 47.1D). (Courtesy of Christine Colton, MD, Rush-Presbyterian-St. Luke's Medical Center, Chicago, Illinois.)

DIAGNOSIS

Primary central nervous system (CNS) lymphoma.

DISCUSSION

Primary CNS lymphoma is an uncommon but increasingly diagnosed tumor that occurs in two different patient populations: immunologically normal patients and immunocompromised patients. The site of origin is unknown since the CNS contains no endogenous lymphoid tissue or lymphatic circulation. Lymphoma in the immunologically normal population typically presents in the sixth decade, whereas AIDS-related disease presents in the fourth decade.

Pathologically, CNS lymphoma can be a circumscribed or a poorly defined infiltrating tumor. It can extend along the perivascular (Virchow-Robin) spaces and infiltrate blood vessel walls. Histologically, one sees small, densely packed neoplastic lymphocytes concentrated in a perivascular pattern.

The classic imaging findings are of a large, rounded-mass lesion involving the deep gray matter, periventricular regions, and/or corpus callosum. Lymphoma is iso- to hyperdense on CT because of its dense cellularity, with homogeneous enhancement. Most lesions are isointense to hypointense to gray matter on T1-weighted images. Lesions are characteristically iso- to slightly hypointense on T2-weighted images, again related to dense cellularity and high nuclear cytoplasmic ratio. Hyperintense lesions can, however, be seen in more necrotic lesions. Seventy-five percent of lesions are in contact with the ependyma, meninges, or both, and most lesions (75% to 85%) are supratentorial. There is usually very little edema relative to lesion size. In approximately 50% of cases, the lesions are multiple. There is typically strong homogeneous enhancement in the immunocompetent population. If there is enhancement along the perivascular spaces, lymphoma should be the number 1 diagnostic consideration, followed by sarcoidosis. Calcification and hemorrhage are uncommon in CNS lymphoma in an immunologically normal patient.

In immunocompromised patients with primary CNS lymphoma, signal characteristics are more heterogeneous and the lesions are typically ring-enhancing because of the higher degree of necrosis in this population. Hemorrhagic lesions are more common, and there is a higher incidence of multifocal disease. Perifocal edema is also reported to be more significant in this population.

Primary CNS lymphoma may present as a diffusely infiltrative lesion without discrete mass lesion. There is involvement of both deep gray matter nuclei and white matter tracts. When there is a "butterfly" pattern of spread across the corpus callosum, discrimination from gliomatosis cerebri is not possible.

In the immunocompromised population, the multifocal enhancing lesions seen in CNS lymphoma are difficult, if not impossible, to distinguish from common opportunistic CNS infections, specifically toxoplasmosis. Differentiation based on imaging criteria is challenging and generally not reliable. The literature highlights some helpful, although not foolproof, imaging clues. A solitary lesion in an immunocompromised patient is more likely to be lymphoma and should carry a lower threshold for biopsy. Toxoplasmosis can, however, present as a solitary lesion (28% to 39%). In general, the average lesion size is larger in lymphoma. Hyperattenuation on noncontrast CT and subependymal spread of tumor have been reported as the most reliable features in the diagnosis of primary CNS lymphoma as opposed to toxoplasmosis in the immunocompromised patient. Thallium radionuclide scanning is very helpful, being positive in lymphoma but not in toxoplasmosis.

Differential diagnosis in the immunocompetent population with primary CNS lymphoma includes glioma, metastasis, and sarcoid. On noncontrast CT the hyperdense lesions can mimic vascular lesions, such as cavernous hemangiomas or arteriovenous malformation.

Primary CNS lymphomas are highly radiosensitive tumors. Most cases regress completely following radiotherapy. Recurrent or progressive disease is common and usually occurs within 1 year. Overall prognosis is poor, with a median survival of 13.5 months after diagnosis.

In contradistinction to primary CNS lymphoma, metastasis to the CNS from systemic lymphoma (or secondary CNS lymphoma) usually manifests as dural or leptomeningeal disease. There may or may not be involvement of the underlying parenchyma.

SUGGESTED READINGS

Baladrishnan J, Becker PS, Kumar AJ, et al. Acquired immunodeficiency syndrome: correlation of radiologic and pathologic findings in the brain. *Radiographics* 1990;10:201–215.

Ciricillo SF, Rosenblum ML. Use of CT and MR imaging to distinguish intracranial lesions and to define the need for biopsy in AIDS patients. *J Neurosurg* 1990;73:720–724.

Dina TS. Primary central nervous system lymphoma versus toxoplasmosis in AIDS. *Radiology* 1991;179:823–828.

Johnson BA, Fram EK, Johnson PC, et al. The variable appearance of primary lymphoma of the central nervous system: comparison with histopathologic features. *AJNR* 1997;18:563–572.

Osborn AG. Meningiomas and other nonglial neoplasms. In: *Diagnostic neuroradiology*. St. Louis: Mosby, 1994:620–622.

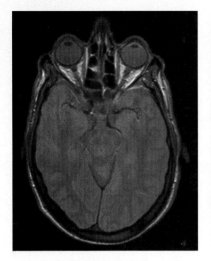

FIGURE 48.1A

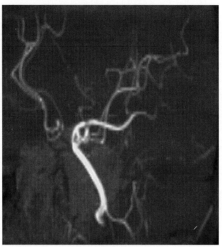

FIGURE 48.1B

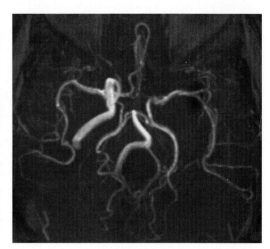

FIGURE 48.1C

CLINICAL HISTORY

An 82-year-old male with transient ischemic attacks.

FINDINGS

Absence of flow void is demonstrated within the cavernous carotid on the proton-density image (Fig. 48.1A) and lack of flow is noted within the petrous, cavernous, and supraclinoid segments of the left carotid artery on the MRA (Fig. 48.1B,C).

DIAGNOSIS

Occlusion or severe stenosis of the left internal carotid artery.

DISCUSSION

Although severe stenosis or occlusion of the intracranial segments of the left internal carotid artery is demonstrated in this case, there is no evidence of infarction of the left cerebral hemisphere because the left anterior and middle cerebral arteries are receiving their blood supply from the right internal carotid artery or the vertebral arteries via the circle of Willis. A complete circle of Willis can be found in approximately 25% of the population.

Submitted by Alan D.S. Chan, MD; William G. Bradley, MD, PhD, FACR (Senior Editor), Long Beach Memorial Medical Center, Long Beach, CA.

SUGGESTED READING

Osborn AG. Diagnostic cerebral angiography. *Stroke.* New York: Lippincott, 1999:395–397.

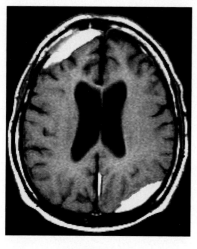

FIGURE 49.1A

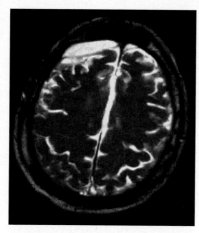

FIGURE 49.1B

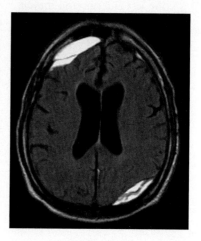

FIGURE 49.1C

CLINICAL HISTORY

A 62-year-old male who presents with altered mental status.

FINDINGS

Axial T1-weighted (Fig. 49.1A), T2-weighted (Fig. 49.1B), and FLAIR (Fig. 49.1C) images demonstrate bilateral subdural collections.

DIAGNOSIS

Bilateral subdural hematomas (coup and contrecoup).

DISCUSSION

Subdural hematomas usually result from tears of bridging cortical veins. The hematomas accumulate in the potential space between the inner dural layer and the arachnoid. They typically spread in a crescentic shape over the cerebral hemispheres without crossing the falx. The subdural collections are hyperintense on both the T1- and T2-weighted images. This MR appearance would suggest that the fluid collections contain subacute, extracellular methemoglobin blood products. The MR appearance of intracranial hemorrhage is divided into hyperacute, acute, subacute, and chronic phases (see table 49.1).

TABLE 49.1

Phase of Hemorrhage	T1-weighted Image	T2-weighted Image	
Hyperacute hemorrhage (<24 hrs)	Isointense	Hyperintense	Oxyhemoglobin (diamagnetic)
Acute hemorrhage (1–3 days)	Isointense	Hypointense	Deoxyhemoglobin (paramagnetic)
Early subacute hemorrhage (4–7 days)	Hyperintense	Hypointense	Intracellular methemoglobin (paramagnetic)
Late subacute hemorrhage (1–2 weeks)	Hyperintense	Hyperintense	Extracellular methemglobin (paramagnetic)
Chronic hemorrhage	Hypointense	Hypointense	Hemosiderin (ferromagnetic)

Submitted by Alan D. S. Chan, MD, William G. Bradley, MD, PhD, FACR (Senior Editor), Long Beach Memorial Medical Center, Long Beach, CA

SUGGESTED READINGS

Evans SJJ, Gean AD. Craniocerebral trauma. In: Stark DD, Bradley WG, eds. *Magnetic resonance imaging,* 3rd ed. St. Louis: Mosby, 1999:1351–1352.

Grossman RI, Yousem DM. *Neuroradiology: the requisites.* St. Louis: Mosby, 1994:176–180.

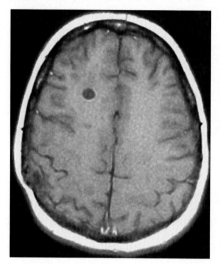

FIGURE 50.1A

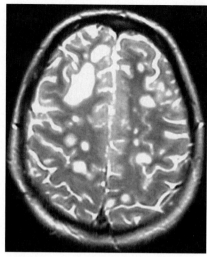

FIGURE 50.1B

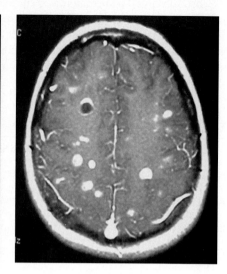

FIGURE 50.1C

CLINICAL HISTORY

A 36-year-old female with history of weakness and paresthesias.

FINDINGS

Axial noncontrast T1-weighted acquisition (Fig. 50.1A) demonstrates a focal, well-defined, round, low-signal lesion within the right centrum semiovale. The T2-weighted image (Fig. 50.1B) shows marked perifocal edema surrounding this lesion. Moreover, there are several additional hyperintense lesions within the deep periventricular and subcortical white matter of both cerebral hemispheres. The T1-weighted image following intravenous contrast (Fig. 50.1C) shows lesion enhancement. (Courtesy of Christine Colton, MD, Rush-Presbyterian-St. Luke's Medical Center, Chicago, Illinois.)

DIAGNOSIS

Necrotizing granulomatous vasculitis.

DISCUSSION

Multifocal, enhancing lesions have a relatively nonspecific appearance, and their finding leads to a relatively wide differential diagnosis, which includes vasculitis. Multiple metastases and demyelinating disease, including multiple sclerosis (MS) and acute disseminated encephalomyelitis (ADEM), are the most common causes. Microangiopathic disease of aging typically does not show foci of enhancement. Multiple venous infarcts are a rare cause of this appearance.

Causes of vasculitis include the idiopathic ones, autoimmune arteritis (which can be associated with the systemic disorders of rheumatoid arthritis, lupus, polyarteritis), primary CNS angiitis, as well as drug-induced conditions (including such recreational drugs as cocaine). Hypertensive encephalopathy can produce a similar MR picture. If CNS vasculitis is clinically suspected and MRI scanning is negative, angiography will almost always be negative as well.

SUGGESTED READINGS

Burger PC, Burch JG, Vogel FS. Granulomatous angiitis. *Stroke* 1977;8:29–35.

Greenan TJ, Grossman RI, Goldberg HI. Cerebral vasculitis: MR imaging and angiographic correlation. *Radiology* 1992;182:65–72.

Llenas JS, Tortella EP. Cerebral angitis. *Neuroradiology* 1978;15:1–11.

Yuh WTC, Ueda T, Maley JE. Perfusion and diffusion imaging: a potential tool for improved diagnosis of CNS vasculitis. *AJNR* 1998;20:87–89.

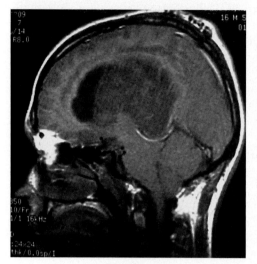

FIGURE 51.1A

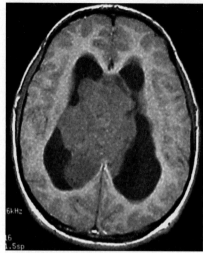

FIGURE 51.1B

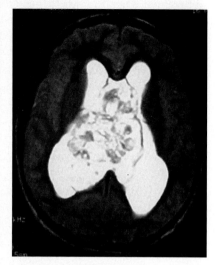

FIGURE 51.1C

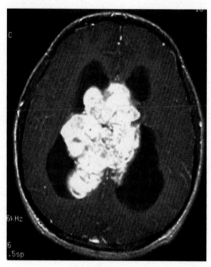

FIGURE 51.1D

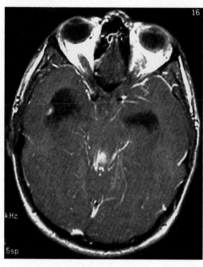

FIGURE 51.1E

CLINICAL HISTORY

A 16-year-old male with history of headaches.

FINDINGS

Sagittal and axial T1-weighted images (Fig. 51.1A,B) demonstrate a large lobulated mass expanding the right and left lateral ventricles centered along the septum pellucidum. There is inferior extension into the region of the enlarged third ventricle with compression upon the optic tracts and chiasm. There is downward transtentorial herniation with compression of the midbrain and brainstem. Additionally, there is tonsillar herniation. The mass is heterogeneous in signal on the T2-weighted acquisition (Fig. 51.1C). Following intravenous contrast (Fig. 51.1D,E), there is heterogeneous enhancement of the intraventricular lesion with tiny nodular regions of enhancement along the ependymal surface of the right lateral ventricle in the region of the antrum and temporal horn.

DIAGNOSIS

Intraventricular pilocytic astrocytoma.

DISCUSSION

One-tenth of all central nervous system (CNS) neoplasms involve the ventricles. Imaging characteristics are nonspecific, and location and patient age become the most helpful information in the differential diagnosis of these lesions.

The differential diagnosis for a lateral ventricular tumor in a child of this age varies according to location within the lateral ventricle. Primitive neuroepithelial tumors (PNET), astrocytomas, and teratomas are the primary considerations for a tumor with its epicenter in the body of the lateral ventricle. Frontal horn tumors include astrocytoma and giant cell astrocytoma, whereas those found in the atrium are usually choroid plexus papillomas, or rarely ependymomas. Tumors are less frequently seen in the temporal and occipital horns. These include meningiomas and enlarged calcified choroid plexi in neurofibromatosis type 2 patients.

Studies have shown peak ages of 2 and 11 years for the occurrence of lateral ventricular tumors. Lateral ventricular tumors are typically bulky lesions associated with hydrocephalus and increased intracranial pressure. In children less than 6 years old, the most common tumors to involve the body of the lateral ventricle are PNET, teratoma, and astrocytoma (usually anaplastic or glioblastoma multiforme). In older children and young adults (seen in this case), astrocytoma is the most common neoplasm to occur in this region. Edema within adjacent brain is an indication of parenchymal invasion and/or a more aggressive (or higher-grade) tumor.

In adults, lateral ventricular tumors involving the body include meningioma, astrocytoma, central neurocytoma, oligodendroglioma, and ependymoma. In addition to these entities, giant cell astrocytoma can be added to the list in frontal horn tumors. Tumors involving the atrium include meningioma and metastases. Meningiomas can rarely be seen in the temporal horn or occipital region of the ventricle.

SUGGESTED READINGS

Duong G, Sarazin L, Bourgouin P, et al. MRI of lateral ventricular tumors. *Can Assoc Radiol J* 1995;46:434–442.

Jelinek J, Smirniotopoulos JG, Parisi JE, et al. Lateral ventricular neoplasms of the brain: differential diagnosis based on clinical, CT, and MR findings. *AJNR* 1990;11:567–574.

Osborn AG. Brain tumors and tumorlike masses: classification and differential diagnosis. In: *Diagnostic neuroradiology*. St. Louis: Mosby, 1994:422–430.

Tien RD. Intraventricular mass lesions of the brain: CT and MR findings. *AJR* 1991;157:1283–1290.

Zuccaro G, Sosa F, Cuccia V. Lateral ventricular tumors in children: a series of 54 cases. *Childs Nerv Syst* 1999;15:774–785.

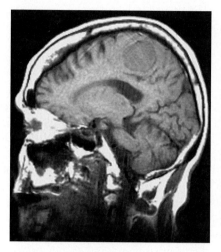

FIGURE 52.1A

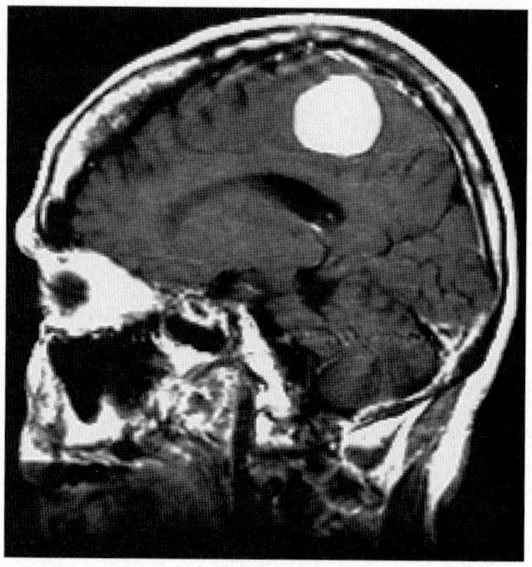

FIGURE 52.1B

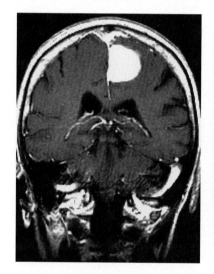

FIGURE 52.1C

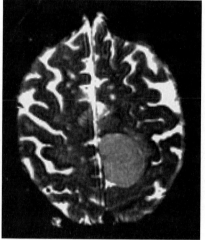

FIGURE 52.1D

CLINICAL HISTORY

A 77-year-old female with headaches and new-onset right leg weakness.

FINDINGS

There is an extraaxial mass arising from the falx in the left frontoparietal region. It demonstrates isointensity on T1-weighted images (Fig. 52.1A) and homogeneous enhancement following administration of gadolinium (Fig. 52.1B,C). Mass effect on the left motor strip is identified, explaining the right leg weakness. Minimal parenchymal edema is noted (Fig. 52.1D).

DIAGNOSIS

Parafalcine meningioma.

DISCUSSION

Meningiomas are the most common extraaxial neoplasm of the brain. There is a preponderance of meningiomas in middle-aged women. Ninety percent occur supratentorially. Other locations include intraosseous and intraventricular (15% third ventricle, 5% fourth ventricle).

Multiple meningiomas occur in the familial syndrome neurofibromatosis type II.

Radiologically on CT, approximately 60% are slightly hyperdense when compared with normal brain tissue, and calcifications are seen in approximately 20% of cases. On contrast CT, there is significant enhancement by meningiomas except in necrotic areas. On MR T1-weighted images demonstrate iso- to slightly hypointensity and T2-weighted images show iso- to hyperintensity relative to normal gray matter. In addition a "dural tail" may be identified, enhancement of the dura trailing off away from the lesion in a crescentic fashion. On angiography, the lesion appears as tumor blush and is known as the "in-law" sign. (The stain comes early and stays late.)

Meningiomas also have associated bony changes in approximately 20% of cases. These include hyperostotic or osteolytic lesions. Meningiomas are also the most common tumor induced by radiation.

Submitted by R. B. Muthyala, MD, University of CA, Irvine Medical Center, Orange, CA; William G. Bradley, MD, PhD, FACR (Senior Editor), Long Beach Memorial Medical Center, Long Beach, CA.

SUGGESTED READINGS

Stock DD, Bradley WG. *Magnetic resonance imaging.* St. Louis: Mosby, 1999.
Grossman D. *Neuroradiology: the requisites.* St. Louis: Mosby, 1994.
Orrison WW. *Neuroimaging.* Philadelphia: WB Saunders, 1998.

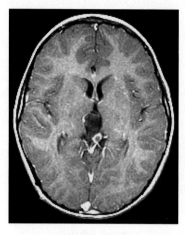

FIGURE 53.1A

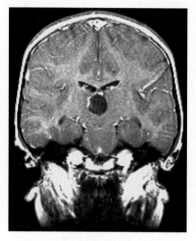

FIGURE 53.1B

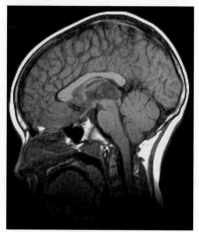

FIGURE 53.1C

CLINICAL HISTORY

A 21-year-old male with recurrent headaches, visual disturbances, and new-onset dizziness.

FINDINGS

A 2-cm mass is present in the pineal region. There is minimal enhancement with contrast (Fig. 53.1A,B). The mass is hypointense on T1-weighted image (Fig. 53.1C).

DIAGNOSIS

Pineocytoma.

DISCUSSION

Pineal region neoplasms are rare, representing only 1% to 3% of all intracranial neoplasms and 3% to 8% of intracranial tumors in children. Clinically, they may present with hydrocephalus (through obstruction of the aqueduct), precocious puberty, or paresis of upward gaze (Parinaud's syndrome).

The normal pineal gland measures about 4 mm in diameter. On MR the normal pineal gland may be visualized as a nodule or a ringlike structure with cysts. Cysts in the pineal gland are noted in 0.6% of children and 2.6% of adults. Calcifications are seen in 11% of children up to age 14 but are generally not noted in children younger than 5 years of age. CT features of pineal tumors include the presence of calcification in young children or abnormal displacement of the calcifications in a normal gland.

Pineal region masses are divided into two categories—those of germ cell origin and those of pineal cell origin. Pineal germ cell tumors include germinomas, teratomas, choriocarcinoma, and endodermal sinus tumors. Germinomas are the most common of pineal tumors and have strong male predominance. On MR germinomas generally demonstrate isointensity to normal brain on T1- and T2-weighted sequences with intense enhancement. Teratomas are the second most common pineal tumor, which also has a strong male predominance. Pineal cell origin tumors include pineocytomas and pineoblastomas. There is an equal gender preponderance, and they account for 15% of pineal region neoplasms.

Pineocytomas account for 11% of pediatric pineal tumors. On MR, findings are nonspecific with hypointensity or isointensity on T1-weighted images and hyperintensity on T2-weighted images. With gadolinium, heterogeneous enhancement is usually present. With regard to pineoblastoma, which tends to be poorly differentiated and highly malignant, MR is also nonspecific, depicting its heterogeneity and heterogeneous enhancement.

Also included in the differential diagnosis are pineal cysts, tectal gliomas and intraventricular masses such as meningiomas, and ependymomas.

Submitted by R.B. Muthyala, University of CA, Irvine Medical Center, Orange, CA; William G. Bradley, MD, PhD, FACR (Senior Editor), Long Beach Memorial Medical Center, Long Beach, CA.

SUGGESTED READINGS

Stock DD, Bradley WG. *Magnetic resonance imaging*. St. Louis: Mosby, 1999.
Orrison WW. *Neuroimaging*. Philadelphia: WB Saunders, 1998.

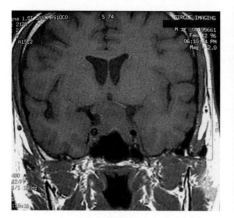

FIGURE 54.1A

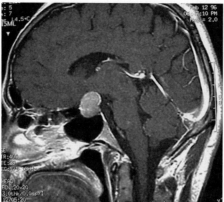

FIGURE 54.1B

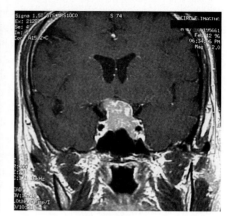

FIGURE 54.1C

CLINICAL HISTORY

A 37-year-old male with visual disturbance.

FINDINGS

Targeted coronal T1-weighted images (Fig. 54.1A) demonstrate a large mass exhibiting intermediate signal within the sella turcica extending cephalad into the suprasellar cistern. The tumor extends into the left cavernous sinus and abuts the cavernous left internal carotid artery (ICA). There is superior displacement of the optic chiasm as well as enlargement of the sella turcica. There is intense homogeneous enhancement following contrast (Fig. 54.1B,C). Note the "snowman" appearance of the mass caused by the "waist" of the diaphragm sella.

DIAGNOSIS

Pituitary macroadenoma.

DISCUSSION

Pituitary adenomas are common lesions, which account for 10% of all intracranial neoplasms. Pituitary tumors are classified by size. Those less than 10 mm are considered microadenomas; those greater than 10 mm are macroadenomas (seen in this case). The clinical presentation of pituitary adenoma depends on the size of the lesion and the presence or absence of hormone production. Twenty-five percent of adenomas are "nonfunctioning" tumors; the remainder show clinical signs of hormone excess. In general, the hormonally active adenomas present earlier in their course of evolution and are typically microadenomas. Macroadenomas are more often "nonfunctioning" and present with signs related to compression or invasion of adjacent structures (i.e., optic chiasm or cavernous sinus). Rarely, an adenoma presents acutely with pituitary apoplexy (severe headache, hypotension, sudden visual loss) because of intratumoral hemorrhage.

Pituitary adenomas are tumors of adults. Fewer than 10% occur in children. Pituitary macroadenoma is the most common suprasellar mass, accounting for 33% to 50% of lesions in this area.

Macroadenomas are isodense on nonenhanced CT, with moderate enhancement. One percent to 8% of lesions calcify. On MRI, uncomplicated macroadenomas are isointense to gray matter on all pulse sequences and enhance following contrast injection. The characteristic configuration seen on coronal and sagittal images is that of a figure-of-eight- or snowman-shaped mass, reflecting an intrasellar mass with suprasellar extension (nicely demonstrated in this case). The "waist" of the lesion is the result of the relative constriction of the mass at the level of the diaphragma sella. Necrosis, cyst formation, and hemorrhage are not uncommon, producing heterogeneous signal. Twenty percent to 30% of adenomas demonstrate hemorrhage. (See Vol I, Case 67.) Infarction and/or hemorrhage, however, rarely produce the clinical syndrome of pituitary apoplexy. Most intratumoral hemorrhage is subclinical and is discovered only incidentally at imaging.

Coronal MRI is best for demonstrating compression and/or invasion of adjacent structures such as the optic chiasm and cavernous sinus. There is often lateral extension of tumor into the region of the cavernous sinus; however, whether there is actually direct invasion of the cavernous sinus is often difficult to determine. Lateral extension and interposition of tumor between the lateral wall of the cavernous sinus and the carotid artery is the most reliable indicator of cavernous sinus invasion. Although cavernous sinus involvement is common, constriction and/or occlusion of the cavernous internal carotid artery is rare. The sphenoid sinus and clivus can also be involved at the time of diagnosis.

Benign invasive pituitary adenoma cannot be differentiated from the rare occurrence of pituitary carcinoma based on imaging features alone.

SUGGESTED READINGS

Elster AD. Modern imaging of the pituitary. *Radiology* 1993;187:1–14.

Johnson DE, Woodruff WW, Allen IS, et al. MR imaging of the sellar and juxtasellar regions. *Radiographics* 1991;11:727–758.

Kucharczyk W, Montanera WJ, Becker LE. The sella turcica and parasellar region. In: Atlas SW, ed. *Magnetic resonance imaging of the brain and spine,* 2nd ed. Philadelphia: Lippincott-Raven, 1996:884–894.

Kyle CA, Laster RA, Burton EM, et al. Subacute pituitary apoplexy: MR and CT appearance. *JCAT* 1990;14:40–44.

Ostrov SG, Quencer RM, Hoffman JC, et al. Hemorrhage within pituitary adenomas: how often associated with pituitary apoplexy syndrome? *AJNR* 1989;10:503–510.

Schwartzberg DG. Imaging of pituitary tumors. *Semin Ultrasound CT MR* 1992;13:207–223.

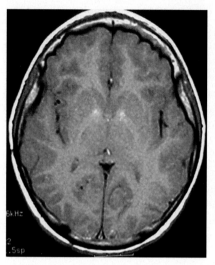

FIGURE 55.1A

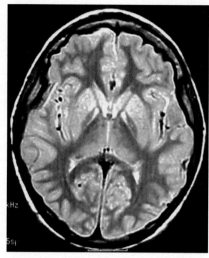

FIGURE 55.1B

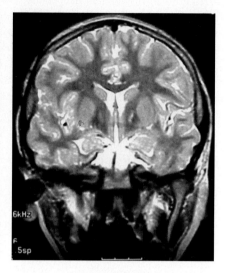

FIGURE 55.1C

CLINICAL HISTORY

A 10-year-old male with history of developmental abnormalities.

FINDINGS

Axial T1-weighted images (Fig. 55.1A) are unremarkable except for small foci of hyperintense signal within the globus pallidus bilaterally. On the axial and coronal T2-weighted images (Fig. 55.1B,C) note the very low signal within the globus pallidus with foci of hyperintense signal centrally, giving a "tiger's eye" appearance. The remainder of the brain appears normal. (Courtesy of Christine Colton, MD, Rush-Presbyterian-St. Luke's Medical Center, Chicago, Illinois.)

DIAGNOSIS

Hallervorden-Spatz disease (HSD).

DISCUSSION

HSD is a rare metabolic disease characterized by progressive neurologic deficits, including gait impairment, rigidity, slowing of voluntary movements, choreoathetosis, dysarthria, dysphasia, optic nerve atrophy, and mental deterioration. Fifty percent of cases are hereditary with autosomal recessive transmission. Onset of symptoms is usually in late adolescence.

Pathologically, there is deposition of iron pigment within the extrapyramidal nuclei (globus pallidus and substantia nigra). There are two types of HSD. Group 1 involves the globus pallidus (GP) and the pars reticulata of the substantia nigra; group 2 involves only the GP. Initially, there is demyelination and reactive gliosis in the involved nuclei, which appear as hyperintense lesions on long TR/TE acquisition. Later in the disease, there is progressive deposition of iron at the periphery of the GP, giving the classic imaging appearance of HSD on T2-weighted image; markedly hypointense GP with small anteromedial foci of high signal ("eye of the tiger" sign). The substantia nigra, if involved, will be hypointense. CT scans show pallidonigral low density.

SUGGESTED READINGS

Angelini L, Nardocci N, Rumi V. Hallervorden-Spatz disease: clinical and magnetic resonance imaging study of 11 cases diagnosed in life. *J Neurol* 1992;239:417–425.

Gallucci M, Cardona F, Arachi M, et al. Follow-up MR studies in Hallervorden-Spatz disease. *JCAT* 1990;14:118–120.

Porter-Grenn L, Sibergliet R, Mehta BA. Hallervorden-Spatz disease with bilateral involvement of globus pallidus and substantia nigra: MR demonstration. *JCAT* 1993;17:961–963.

Savolardo M, Halliday WC, Nardocci N, et al. Hallervorden-Spatz disease: MR and pathologic findings. *AJNR* 1993;14:155–162.

Sethi KD, Adams RJ, Lorring DW, et al. Hallervorden-Spatz disease: clinical and magnetic resonance imaging correlation. *Ann Neurol* 1988;24:692–694.

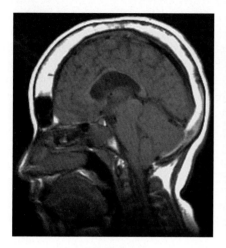

FIGURE 56.1A

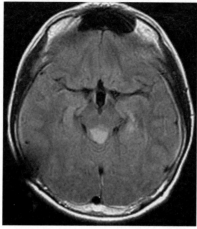

FIGURE 56.1B

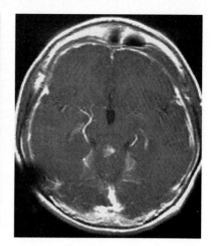

FIGURE 56.1C

CLINICAL HISTORY

A 20-year-old female with history of visual disturbance and chronic headaches.

FINDINGS

There is a 1.5-cm tectal mass. On the T1-weighted sagittal image, the mass appears isointense to brain (Fig. 56.1A). On the axial FLAIR image (Fig. 56.1B), the lesion appears hyperintense to brain tissue. The mass enhances with gadolinium, as seen on the axial image in Fig. 56.1B. Metallic artifact is noted in the posterior right temporal region from a shunt reservoir. Diffuse meningeal enhancement is seen.

DIAGNOSIS

Tectal glioma with benign meningeal fibrosis from chronic shunting.

DISCUSSION

The tectum ("roof") is the portion of the midbrain posterior to the cerebral aqueduct and consists of the quadrigeminal plate (i.e., the superior and inferior colliculi). Tectal gliomas have an equal male, female gender preference and generally present with aqueductal obstruction and hydrocephalus.

On MRI, tectal gliomas are generally isointense to brain on T1-weighted images and slightly hyperintense on T2-weighted or FLAIR images. Enhancement is variable and calcification is rare.

Differential diagnosis includes pineal masses (i.e., those of pineal cell origin such as pineoblastomas and pineocytoma), and those of germ cell origin, such as germinoma, choriocarcinoma, endodermal cell carcinoma, and teratoma. Benign pineal cysts, cavernous hemangiomas, and meningiomas are also possible in this area.

Benign meningeal fibrosis is probably due to bleeding between the leaves of the dura with secondary inflammation.

Submitted by R.B. Muthyala, MD, University of CA, Irvine Medical Center, Orange, CA; William G. Bradley, MD, PhD, FACR (Senior Editor), Long Beach Memorial Medical Center, Long Beach, CA.

SUGGESTED READINGS

Grossman R. *Neuroradiology: the requisites* St. Louis: Mosby, 1994.
Russell DS. *Pathology of tumours of the nervous system,* 5th ed. Baltimore: Williams & Wilkins, 1989.

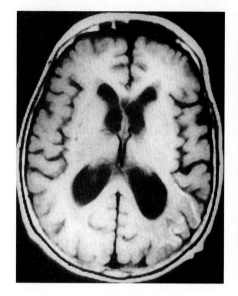

FIGURE 57.1A

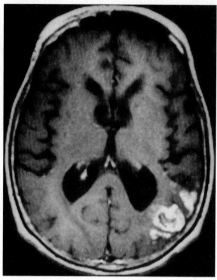

FIGURE 57.1B

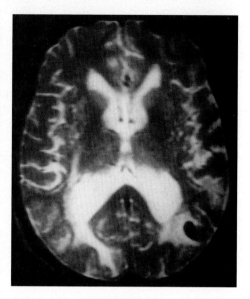

FIGURE 57.1C

CLINICAL HISTORY

A 68-year-old female with acute onset of aphasia 2 weeks previously.

FINDINGS

T1-weighted axial image demonstrates subtle, left parietal gyral hyperintensity (Fig. 57.1A) that enhances following administration of gadolinium (Fig. 57.1B). On a T2-weighted image through the same level (Fig. 57.1C), this area turns hypointense.

DIAGNOSIS

Subacute cortical infarct.

DISCUSSION

Infarcts can be staged as acute, subacute, and chronic, based on their mass effect and the presence of gyral hyperintensity on T1-weighted images and enhancement following administration of gadolinium. During the acute phase (0 to 10 days), mass effect is present but there is no evidence of petechial hemorrhage in gyri, nor is there evidence of gadolinium enhancement. By the subacute phase (10 days to 3 months), there is no evidence of significant mass effect or atrophy and petechial hemorrhage is noted in the gyri, which enhance with gadolinium. In the chronic stage (more than 3 months), atrophy is present and there may be persistence of the gyral hyperintensity on a T1-weighted image; however, there is usually minimal enhancement.

The inherent gyral signal abnormality on the T1- (Fig. 57.1A) and T2-weighted (Fig. 57.1C) images is consistent with intracellular methemoglobin. There may be a component of laminar necrosis. The gyral enhancement in the subacute stage is indicative of loss of autoregulation and blood-brain barrier breakdown.

Submitted by William G. Bradley, MD, PhD, FACR (Senior Editor), Long Beach Memorial Medical Center, Long Beach, CA.

SUGGESTED READING

Jensen MC, Brant-Zawadzki MN, Jacobs BC. Ischemia. In: Stark DD, Bradley WG, eds. *Magnetic resonance imaging,* 3rd ed. St. Louis: Mosby, 1999:1255–1276.

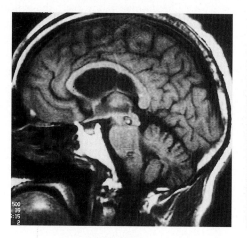

FIGURE 58.1A

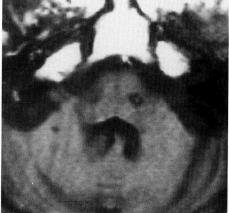

FIGURE 58.1B

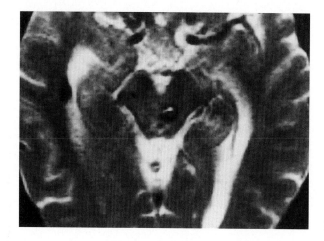

FIGURE 58.1C

CLINICAL HISTORY

A 39-year-old Hispanic male with chronic left third nerve palsy and seizures.

FINDINGS

T1- and T2-weighted axial and sagittal images (Fig. 58.1A–C) demonstrate hyperintense lesions in the brainstem with the surrounding hypointense borders.

DIAGNOSIS

Multiple cavernous angiomas.

DISCUSSION

Rigamonti et al. first described the syndrome of multiple cavernous angiomas in the Hispanic population. However, it has now been seen in all ethnic groups. The disease is frequently familial and may be asymptomatic. When symptomatic, the patients usually present with seizures due to cortical involvement. In addition to seizures, this patient had a left third nerve palsy due to the lesion position just anterior to the left third nerve nucleus (Fig. 58.1C).

Cavernous angiomas tend to continue to bleed into their sinusoids, forming a mulberry lesion consisting of central methemoglobin with peripheral hemosiderin with rounded mass effect. (This is in contradistinction to other parenchymal hemorrhages, which generally resolve to the hemosiderin line slit without mass effect.)

Whereas the syndrome of multiple cavernous angiomas seems to be familial (and therefore genetically determined), the occurrence of isolated cavernous angiomas appears to be the result of a different mechanism, often originating from a venous angioma.

High-field gradient-echo images are the most sensitive to detect the hemosiderin resulting from bleeding of these lesions, if they are suspected clinically.

Cavernous angiomas are generally only treated surgically following hemorrhage large enough to compromise vital structures (i.e., usually in the posterior fossa).

Submitted by William G. Bradley, MD, PhD, FACR (Senior Editor), Long Beach Memorial Medical Center, Long Beach, CA.

SUGGESTED READINGS

Bradley WG. Brainstem: normal anatomy and pathology. In: Stark DD, Bradley WG, eds. *Magnetic resonance imaging,* 3rd ed. St. Louis: Mosby, 1999:1187–1208.

Bradley WG. Hemorrhage. In: Stark DD, Bradley WG, eds. *Magnetic resonance imaging,* 3rd ed. St. Louis: Mosby, 1999:1329–1346.

Dillon WP. Cryptic vascular malformations: controversies in terminology, diagnosis, pathophysiology, and treatment. *AJNR* 1997;18:1839–1846.

Rigamonti D, Hadley MN, Drayer BP, et al. Cerebral cavernous malformations: incidence and familial occurrence. *N Engl J Med* 1988;11:319:343–347.

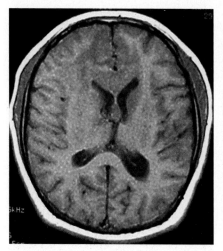

FIGURE 59.1A

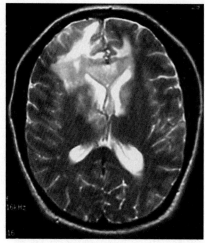

FIGURE 59.1B

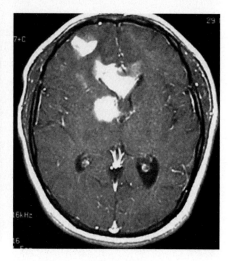

FIGURE 59.1C

CLINICAL HISTORY

A 29-year-old male with history of personality change. The patient had prior lymphoma of the femur.

FINDINGS

Axial T1- and T2-weighted images (Fig. 59.1A,B) demonstrate abnormal signal in the head of the caudate nuclei bilaterally extending into the frontal lobes. There is extension of signal abnormality across the genu of the corpus callosum as well as thickening of the septum pellucidum. The lesion is hypointense on the T1-weighted acquisition and iso- to slightly hyperintense on T2-weighted images. Perifocal edema is seen within the subcortical white matter of the frontal lobes bilaterally. Following intravenous contrast on the T1-weighted image (Fig. 59.1C), there is intense globular enhancement within the right basal ganglia, subcortical white matter of the right frontal lobe, and corpus callosum.

DIAGNOSIS

Central nervous system (CNS) lymphoma.

DISCUSSION

Primary CNS lymphoma is an uncommon but increasingly diagnosed tumor that occurs in two different patient populations: immunologically normal patients and immunocompromised patients. The site of origin is unknown since the CNS contains no endogenous lymphoid tissue or lymphatic circulation. Lymphoma in the immunologically normal population typically presents in the sixth decade, whereas AIDS-related disease presents in the fourth decade.

Pathologically, CNS lymphoma can be a circumscribed or a poorly defined infiltrating tumor. It can extend along the perivascular (Virchow-Robin) spaces and infiltrate blood vessel walls. On histologic examination, one sees small, densely packed neoplastic lymphocytes concentrated in a perivascular pattern.

The classic imaging finding is that of a large, rounded-mass lesion involving the deep gray matter, periventricular regions, and/or corpus callosum. Lymphoma is iso- to hyperdense on CT due to its dense cellularity, with homogeneous enhancement. Most lesions are isointense to hypointense to gray matter on T1-weighted images. Lesions are characteristically iso- to slightly hypointense on T2-weighted images, again related to dense cellularity and high nuclear cytoplasmic ratio. Hyperintense lesions can, however, be seen in more necrotic lesions. Seventy-five percent of lesions are in contact with the ependyma, meninges, or both, and most lesions (75% to 85%) are supratentorial. There is usually very little edema relative to lesion size. In approximately 50% of cases, the lesions are multiple. There is typically strong homogeneous enhancement in the immunocompetent population. If there is enhancement along the perivascular spaces, lymphoma should be the number 1 diagnostic consideration, followed by sarcoidosis. Calcification and hemorrhage are uncommon in CNS lymphoma in an immunologically normal patient.

In immunocompromised patients with primary CNS lymphoma, signal characteristics are more heterogeneous and the lesions are typically ring enhancing because of the higher degree of necrosis in this population. Hemorrhagic lesions are more common and there is a higher incidence of multifocal disease. Perifocal edema is also reported to be more significant in this population.

Primary CNS lymphoma may present as a diffusely infiltrative lesion without discrete mass lesion. There is involvement of both deep gray matter nuclei and white matter tracts. When there is a "butterfly" pattern of spread (as seen in this case) across the corpus callosum, discrimination from gliomatosis cerebri is not possible.

In the immunocompromised population, the multifocal enhancing lesions seen in CNS lymphoma are difficult, if not impossible, to distinguish from common opportunistic CNS infections, specifically toxoplasmosis. Differentiation based on imaging criteria is challenging and generally not reliable. The literature highlights some helpful, although not foolproof, imaging clues. A solitary lesion in an immunocompromised patient is more likely to be lymphoma and should carry a lower threshold for biopsy. Toxoplasmosis can, however, present as a solitary lesion (28% to 39%). In general, the average lesion size is larger in lymphoma. Hyperattenuation on noncontrast CT and the presence of subependymal spread of tumor have been reported as the most reliable features in the diagnosis of primary CNS lymphoma as opposed to toxoplasmosis in the immunocompromised patient. Thallium radionuclide scanning is very helpful, being positive in lymphoma but not in toxoplasmosis.

Differential diagnosis in the immunocompetent population with primary CNS lymphoma includes glioma, metastasis, and sarcoid. On noncontrast CT the hyperdense lesions can mimic vascular lesions, such as cavernous hemangiomas or arteriovenous malformation.

Primary CNS lymphomas are highly radiosensitive tumors. Most cases regress completely following radiotherapy. Recurrent or progressive disease is common and usually occurs within 1 year. Overall prognosis is poor with a median survival of 13.5 months after diagnosis.

In contradistinction to primary CNS lymphoma, metastasis to the CNS from systemic lymphoma (or secondary CNS lymphoma) usually manifests as dural or leptomeningeal disease. There may or may not be involvement of the underlying parenchyma.

SUGGESTED READINGS

Baladrishnan J, Becker PS, Kumar AJ, et al. Acquired immunodeficiency syndrome: correlation of radiologic and pathologic findings in the brain. *Radiographics* 1990;10:201–215.

Ciricillo SF, Rosenblum ML. Use of CT and MR imaging to distinguish intracranial lesions and to define the need for biopsy in AIDS patients. *J Neurosurg* 1990;73:720–724.

Dina TS. Primary central nervous system lymphoma versus toxoplasmosis in AIDS. *Radiology* 1991;179:823–828.

Johnson BA, Fram EK, Johnson PC, et al. The variable appearance of primary lymphoma of the central nervous system: comparison with histopathologic features. *AJNR* 1997;18:563–572.

Osborn AG. Meningiomas and other nonglial neoplasms. In: *Diagnostic neuroradiology*. St. Louis: Mosby, 1994:620–622.

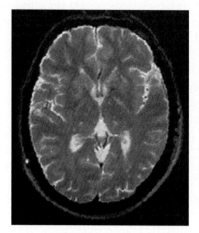

FIGURE 60.1A

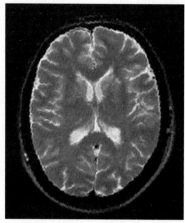

FIGURE 60.1B

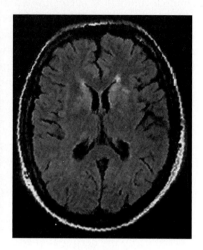

FIGURE 60.1C

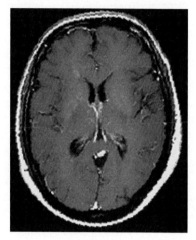

FIGURE 60.1D

CLINICAL HISTORY

A 31-year-old HIV-positive male with headaches.

FINDINGS

Axial T2-weighted and FLAIR images show dilated perivascular (Virchow Robin) spaces in the basal ganglia bilaterally (Fig. 60.1A–C). No significant enhancement is evident following gadolinium administration on T1-weighted images (Fig. 60.1D).

DIAGNOSIS

Cryptococcal meningitis.

DISCUSSION

Cryptococcus neoformans is an opportunistic fungal infection that affects immunocompromised patients, especially those with AIDS or organ transplants.

Cryptococcal meningitis has a tendency to involve the basal meninges, where enhancement can be seen in approximately 30% of cases. It also tends to spread along the perivascular spaces of the lenticulostriate and thalamoperforator arteries. This results in apparent dilation of the perivascular spaces due to characteristic gelatinous pseudocysts, which are typically isointense to cerebrospinal fluid (i.e., hyperintense on T2-weighted images and hypointense on T1-weighted images, without enhancement).

Submitted by Sattam Lingawi, MB, ChB, FRCPC; Peter Brotchie, MBBS, PhD; William G. Bradley, MD, PhD, FACR (Senior Editor), Long Beach Memorial Medical Center, Long Beach, CA.

SUGGESTED READINGS

Berkefeld J, Enzensberger W, Lanfermann H. Cryptococcus meningoencephalitis in AIDS: parenchymal and meningeal forms. *Neuroradiology* 1999;41:129–133.

Miszkiel KA. The spectrum of MRI findings in CNS cryptococcosis in AIDS. *Clin Radiol* 1996;51:842–850.

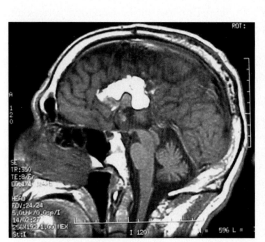

FIGURE 61.1A

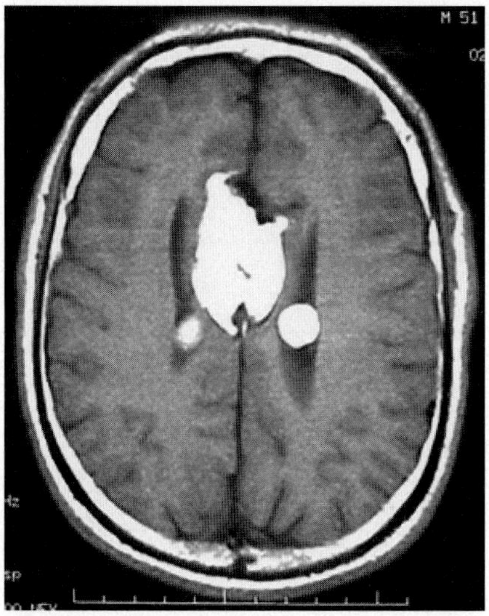

FIGURE 61.1B

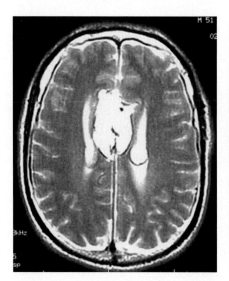

FIGURE 61.1C

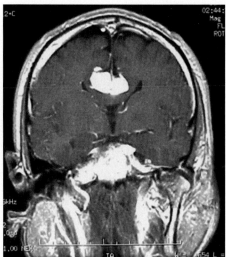

FIGURE 61.1D

CLINICAL HISTORY

A 51-year-old male with headaches.

FINDINGS

Midline sagittal and axial noncontrast T1-weighted images (Fig. 61.1A,B) show dysgenesis of the corpus callosum. Only a portion of the genu of the corpus callosum is identified. There is a large lobulated hyperintense mass in the expected location of the corpus callosum with extension into the posterior lateral ventricles. Note the parallel configuration of the lateral ventricles on the axial acquisition. The mass remains hyperintense on the fast spin-echo

T2-weighted image (Fig. 61.1C). Note chemical shift artifact in the frequency-encoded (anteroposterior) direction. Following intravenous contrast (Fig. 61.1D), there is no significant enhancement of the mass on the T1-weighted image. Also note the "steer head" configuration of the lateral and third ventricles in the coronal plane, a characteristic finding in callosal dysgenesis.

DIAGNOSIS

Corpus callosum dysgenesis with pericallosal lipoma.

DISCUSSION

Intracranial lipomas are malformations related to abnormal differentiation of the meninx primitiva, an undifferentiated mesenchyme that surrounds the developing brain. The meninx primitiva normally develops into the leptomeninges and subarachnoid space. Sometimes, for unknown reasons, the meninx primitiva will differentiate into fat, resulting in an intracranial lipoma. Because of their origin from the meninx (a leptomeninges precursor), lipomas typically arise in or near the subarachnoid space. Intracranial lipomas are considered malformations as opposed to neoplasms and therefore do not grow. They can, however, hypertrophy when a patient gains weight, just like other fat cells in the body. Lipomas almost never exert mass effect and typically have normal structures passing through them, such as blood vessels and cranial nerves. In light of this fact, surgical excision has a high morbidity and is contraindicated.

The most common locations for intracranial lipoma are the deep interhemispheric fissure (40% to 50%), the quadrigeminal plate/supracerebellar cistern (20% to 30%), the suprasellar cistern/interpeduncular cistern (10% to 20%), the cerebellopontine angle cistern (10%), and the Sylvian cistern (5%). Encephaloceles and cutaneous lipomas (usually in the frontal region) may also be present. Many of the midline developmental anomalies have an interhemispheric lipoma as a part of the syndrome.

Interhemispheric lipomas are often associated with hypogenesis or agenesis of the corpus callosum. There are two types of callosal lipoma: the large (more than 2 cm) anteriorly situated tubulonodular type that is typically associated with callosal dysgenesis (seen in this case) and the more posterior thin, curvilinear (C-shaped) lipoma, which curves around the splenium of the corpus callosum. The callosum in these cases is usually normal or near normal. (There may be thinning or shortening of corpus.)

Neuroimaging demonstrates a sharply circumscribed, markedly hypodense mass on CT. Peripheral curvilinear or central nodular calcification is often present. The extent of callosal dysgenesis is best evaluated on MRI. Lipomas are hyperintense on T1-weighted images, becoming less intense on progressively longer time to echo (TE) images. Large lipomas can show "chemical shift" artifact related to differences in resonant frequencies of water and fat protons. This is nicely demonstrated in this case as a region of signal void at the fat-water interface and hyperintensity at water-fat interface, along the frequency encoded axis. Small lipomas may not show a discernible "chemical shift" artifact. Fat suppression techniques can also help identify lipomas by making the fat isointense to gray matter.

SUGGESTED READINGS

Barkovich AJ. Congenital malformations of the brain and skull. In: *Pediatric neuroimaging*, 2nd ed. Philadelphia: Lippincott-Raven, 1996:190.

Dean B, Drayer BP, Beresini DC. MR imaging of pericallosal lipoma. *AJNR* 1988;9:929–931.

Tart RP, Quisling RG. Curvilinear and tubulonodular varieties of lipoma of the corpus callosum: an MR and CT study. *JCAT* 1991;15:805–810.

Truit CL, Barkovich AJ. Pathogenesis of intracranial lipoma: an MR study in 42 patients. *AJNR* 1990;155:855–864.

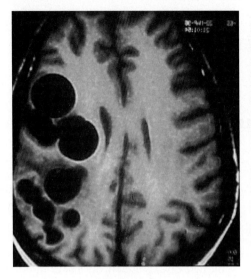 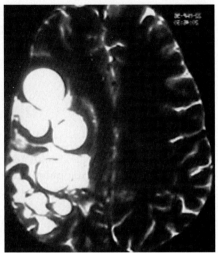

FIGURE 62.1A   **FIGURE 62.1B**

CLINICAL HISTORY

A 30-year-old East Indian male with seizures.

FINDINGS

Axial T1- and T2-weighted images (Fig. 62.1A,B) demonstrate multiple well-defined cystic masses within the right posterior frontal and parietal lobes. There is mild effacement of the body of the right lateral ventricle with slight shift of the midline structures to the left. Mild perilesional high signal is seen on the T2-weighted image consistent with edema. (Courtesy of Tufail Patankar, MD, Manchester, England.)

DIAGNOSIS

Central nervous system (CNS) hydatid disease.

DISCUSSION

Echinococcus granulosus is the primary pathogen responsible for CNS hydatid disease. *Echinococcus multilocularis* may also infest the brain. Hydatid disease is an endemic disease encountered in the Middle East, South America, Australia, and countries surrounding the Mediterranean Sea. It is an unusual disease, accounting for only 2% of intracranial mass lesions, even in endemic areas.

Echinococcus is a tapeworm that lives in the gastrointestinal tract of mammals. The eggs are passed into the feces of the definitive host and ingested by the intermediate host (most often sheep but also humans). The organism penetrates the intestinal wall and spreads via vascular channels and lymphatics. The typical end organs are the liver and lung, with occasional involvement of the brain. Here the parasite enters the larval stage and forms a slowly enlarging cyst. In *E. multilocularis* infestation, clusters of small, grapelike cysts can be seen (known as alveolar echinococcosis).

Clinical presentation is usually related to mass effect of the cyst. Symptoms typically occur late because of the cyst's slow growth. Signs and symptoms include nausea, headache, vomiting, seizures, papilledema, hemiparesis, and cranial nerve palsies.

Pathologic examination shows that the cysts are composed of an inner layer, the endocyst, which is formed by the organism itself and an outer layer, or ectocyst, which is composed of glial tissue and is formed by the host response to the lesion. Echinococcal cysts typically enlarge by 1 to 5 mm per year.

The CT features include a large, thin-walled, unilocular cyst, which follows cerebrospinal fluid (CSF) density. There is local mass effect but no edema or enhancement. Calcification may be seen in the cyst wall or within internal septations. Peripheral masses may demonstrate remodeling of the overlying calvarium. On MRI, echinococcal cysts are hyperintense to CSF on T1- and PD-weighted images and isointense on T2-weighted images. There is typically no surrounding edema or enhancement. Cysts are usually parenchymal, most commonly involving the parietal lobe. Subarachnoid cysts have been reported. Contrast enhancement and edema have been described in the smaller, multiloculated (alveolar) form of disease (*E. multilocularis* disease).

SUGGESTED READINGS

Demir K, Karsli AF, Kaya T, et al. Cerebral hydatid cysts: CT appearance. *Neurology* 1991;33:22–24.

Falcone S, Quencer RM, Post MJD. Magnetic resonance imaging of unusual intracranial infections. *Topic Magn Reson Imag* 1994;6:41–52.

Tsitouridis J, Dimitriadis AS, Kazana E. MRI in cisternal hydatid cysts. *AJNR* 1997;18:1586–1587.

Tunaci M, Tunaci A, Engin G, et al. MRI of cerebral alveolar echinococcosis. *Neuroradiology* 1999;41:844–846.

Tuzin M, Hekimoglu B. Hydatid disease of the CNS: imaging features. *AJR* 1998;171:1497–1450.

Von Sinner W, te Strake L, Clark D. MR imaging in hydatid disease. *AJR* 1991;157:741–745.

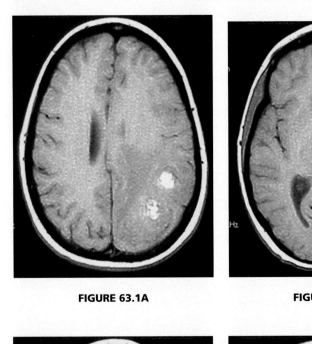

FIGURE 63.1A

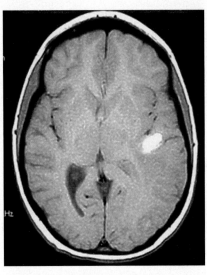

FIGURE 63.1B

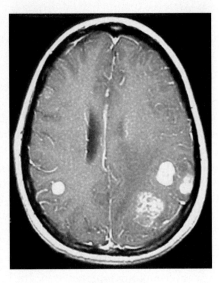

FIGURE 63.1C

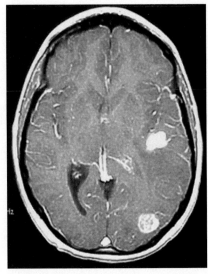

FIGURE 63.1D

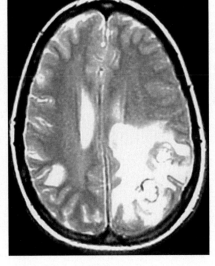

FIGURE 63.1E

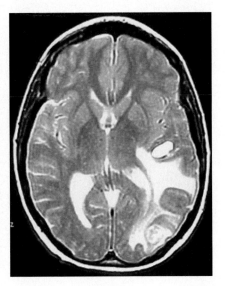

FIGURE 63.1F

CLINICAL HISTORY

A 29-year-old female who at 5 weeks of pregnancy develops severe headaches, nausea, and vomiting.

FINDINGS

Axial pre- and postcontrast T1-weighted images at similar levels (Fig. 63.1A–D) show multiple heterogeneously enhancing masses primarily at the corticomedullary junction of both cerebral hemispheres. A dura-based lesion is seen within the left parietal lobe. Most of these lesions are hyperintense in the noncontrast T1-weighted acquisition consistent with hemorrhage. There is significant perilesional edema, as seen on the axial T2-weighted images (Fig. 63.1E,F), with effacement of overlying cortical sulci as well as effacement of the left lateral ventricle and shift of the midline structures toward the right. (Courtesy of Christine Colton, MD, Rush-Presbyterian-St. Luke's Medical Center, Chicago, Illinois.)

DIAGNOSIS

Hemorrhagic metastases—melanoma.

DISCUSSION

Metastatic tumor to the brain typically occurs via hematogenous spread of tumor from an extracranial site, or occasionally by direct extension from skull metastases or nasopharyngeal routes. Hematogenous metastases may deposit in the brain parenchyma, dura, or calvarium. The primary tumors that most frequently metastasize to the brain are lung, breast, skin (melanoma), gastrointestinal, and genitourinary neoplasms. In adults, cerebral metastases are common, representing 25% to 35% of all brain tumors. In more than 80% of cases, parenchymal metastases are multifocal; however, solitary metastases do occur (30% to 50%), usually from lung, breast, or melanoma primaries. All areas of the brain can be affected, but the corticomedullary junction is the most common site. This is related to the dramatic narrowing of the diameter of the arterioles that supply the cortex in this region. Fewer than 20% of metastases are hemorrhagic; these include choriocarcinoma, renal cell, melanoma, and thyroid carcinomas.

Clinically, parenchymal metastases range from asymptomatic (usually lung cancer or melanoma) to severe neurologic deficit.

Imaging features vary with the type of primary neoplasm. On CT, metastases are typically isodense. There is usually striking perilesional edema, greater than expected for lesion size. The hypodense edema may be the only abnormality identified on noncontrast CT scan. Hyperdense metastases are seen with hemorrhagic metastases, small round cell tumors (lymphoma), and mucinous tumors (gastrointestinal adenocarcinoma). Most metastases enhance strongly following contrast on CT, exhibiting a solid or ringlike pattern. False-negative studies occur in 11.5% of patients on CT if scanned immediately following administration of the standard contrast dose. Double-dose, delayed imaging has been shown to improve the sensitivity and specificity for detecting parenchymal metastatic disease on CT.

MRI with contrast is the most sensitive imaging modality in the detection of central nervous system (CNS) metastases. Signal intensity is variable. Most nonhemorrhagic lesions are hypointense on T1-weighted images and hyperintense on T2-weighted images. In metastatic melanoma with high melanin content or hemorrhage, lesions are typically hyperintense on T1-weighted acquisition and iso- to hypointense on T2-weighted images. This finding, however, is not common, as most melanoma is either amelanotic or has low melanin content. Most melanoma will demonstrate prolonged T1 and T2 signal characteristics unless hemorrhagic (which is common in such metastases). Mucinous adenocarcinoma (typically colon) and densely cellular tumors with high nuclear/cytoplasmic ratios (including lymphoma) may also be hypointense on T2-weighted images. Hemorrhagic metastases have complex imaging characteristics, which depend on the stage of degradation of blood products. In the late stage, a hemosiderin ring may be present.

Typically, a significant amount of perilesional edema is associated with metastases relative to lesion size. The edema pattern on PD, T2, and FLAIR images follows the white matter tracts with sparing of the overlying cortex due to changes in vascular permeability (vasogenic edema pattern). Edema does not typically cross the corpus callosum or involve the cortex, which helps differentiate metastases from primary brain tumor. Cortical metastases do occur. They typically elicit very little perilesional edema, probably due to very little surrounding interstitium.

The vast majority of lesions enhance following contrast in a solid, rim, or nodular pattern. High dose contrast (0.3 mmol/kg) has been shown to be even more sensitive in the detection of CNS metastases, particularly in the evaluation of small lesions, additional lesions, and early disease.

The differential diagnosis for multiple parenchymal enhancing lesions in the brain includes metastases, vasculitis, embolic infarcts, demyelinating disease, abscesses, multifocal glioma, and radiation necrosis. For a solitary enhancing supratentorial lesion, glioblastoma multiforme, abscess, and metastases are the primary diagnostic considerations. In the posterior fossa, a solitary lesion could be metastases, hemangioblastoma, or lymphoma.

SUGGESTED READINGS

Atlas SW, Grossman RI, Gomori JM, et al. MR imaging of intracranial metastatic melanoma. *JCAT* 1987;11:577–582.

Atlas SW, Lavi E. Intra-axial brain tumors. In: Atlas SW, ed., *Magnetic resonance imaging of the brain and spine*, 2nd ed. Philadelphia: Lippincott-Raven 1996:407–415.

Davis PC, Hudgins PA, Peterman SB, et al. Diagnosis of cerebral metastases: double-dose delayed CT vs. contrast-enhanced MR imaging. *AJNR* 1991;12:293–300.

Destian S, Sze G, Krol G, et al. MR imaging of hemorrhagic intracranial neoplasms. *AJR* 1989;152:137–144.

Egelhoff JC, Ross JS, Modic MT, et al. MR imaging of metastatic GI adenocarcinoma in brain. *AJNR* 1992;13:1221–1224.

Haustein J, Laniado M, Neindorf H-P, et al. Triple-dose versus standard-dose gadopentetate dimeglumine: a randomized study in 199 patients. *Radiology* 1993;186:855–860.

Isiklar I, Leeds NE, Fuller GN, et al. Intracranial metastatic melanoma: correlation between MR imaging characteristics and melanin content. *AJR* 1995;165:1503–1512.

Osborn AG. Miscellaneous tumors, cysts, and metastases. In: *Diagnostic neuroradiology*. St. Louis: Mosby, 1994:660–665.

Runge VM, Wells JD, Williams NM. MR imaging of an experimental model of intracranial metastatic disease. A study of lesion detection. *Invest Radiol* 1994;29:1050–1056.

Yuh WTC, Engelken JD, Muhonen MG, et al. Experience with high-dose gadolinium MR imaging in the evaluation of brain metastases. *AJNR* 1992;13:335–345.

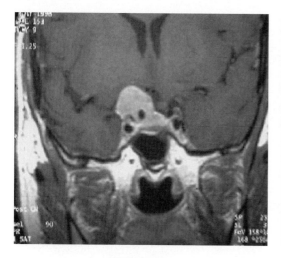

FIGURE 64.1A

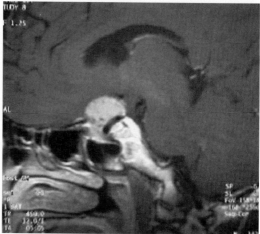

FIGURE 64.1B

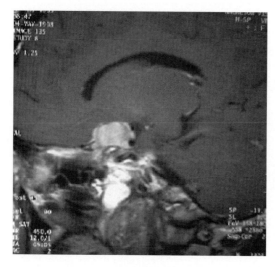

FIGURE 64.1C

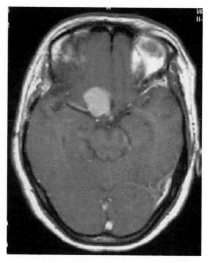

FIGURE 64.1D

CLINICAL HISTORY

A 42-year-old female with gradually developing right eye blindness.

FINDINGS

T1-weighted images with gadolinium (Fig. 64.1A–D) show a homogeneously enhancing mass on the right planum sphenoidale extending into the right parasellar region. There is extension of the mass to the superior wall of the sphenoid sinus and the right side of the optic chiasm with encasement of the right supraclinoid internal carotid artery.

DIAGNOSIS

Planum sphenoidale meningioma.

DISCUSSION

Contrast enhancement provides useful additional information in characterizing brain tumors, including meningiomas. It provides better definition of tumor extent as seen in this example. Fat-suppressed enhanced T1-weighted images are helpful in delineating subtle extension into the orbit or cavernous sinus. Typically, meningiomas display strong diffuse enhancement and are isointense or slightly hypointense on T1-weighted images before contrast. An idea of the histologic subtype can be obtained from signal changes and the severity of edema (if present). Angioplastic and syncytial subtypes are generally hyperintense on T2-weighted images and can be associated with significant edema. Transitional and fibroblastic subtypes tend to be slightly iso- or hypointense on T1- and T2-weighted images. If present, surrounding edema tends to be mild. The differential diagnosis of a meningioma in the suprasellar region includes craniopharyngioma, hypothalamic glioma, thrombosed aneurysm, and pituitary macroadenoma. Hyperostosis can be seen with sphenoidal meningiomas. Meningiomas occur predominantly in females and are frequently seen incidentally in elderly patients. The strong contrast enhancement is due to the large vascular supply by meningeal vessels. However, with larger tumors, cerebral vessels also contribute to the blood supply.

Submitted by Hesham Sabir, MB, ChB; Sattam Lingawi, MB, ChB, FRCPC; Peter Brotchie, MBBS, PhD; William G. Bradley, MD, PhD, FACR (Senior Editor), Long Beach Memorial Medical Center, Long Beach, CA.

SUGGESTED READING

Zee CS. Magnetic resonance imaging of meningiomas. *Semin Ultrasound CT MRI* 1992;13:154–169.

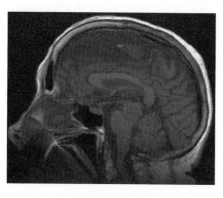

FIGURE 65.1A

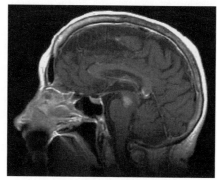

FIGURE 65.1B

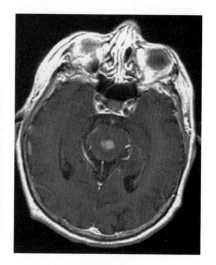

FIGURE 65.1C

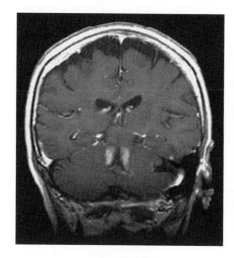

FIGURE 65.1D

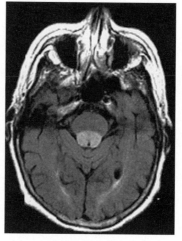

FIGURE 65.1E

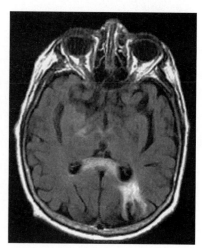

FIGURE 65.1F

CLINICAL HISTORY

An 80-year-old alcoholic female with sudden onset of confusion and ataxia.

FINDINGS

T1-weighted images demonstrate low signal in the midbrain with enhancement in the periaqueductal gray matter following administration of gadolinium (Fig. 65.1A–C). Enhancement is also evident along the undersurface of the splenium of the corpus callosum (Fig. 65.1B). FLAIR images demonstrate hyperintensity along the periaqueductal gray matter and within the splenium (Fig. 65.1E,F).

DIAGNOSIS

Wernicke encephalopathy.

DISCUSSION

Wernicke encephalopathy has also been referred to as *polioencephalitis hemorrhagica superior*. It is an acute or subacute disorder that results from a thiamine deficiency that occurs commonly but not exclusively in alcoholics. It is characterized by the triad of ophthalmoplegia, ataxia, and confusion.

Wernicke-Korsakoff syndrome is a variant condition in which the patient has loss of short-term memory and develops a psychosis in the form of confabulations. In severe cases this condition may be associated with insomnia, cognitive decline, confusion, stupor, and ultimately coma.

On MRI, T2 hyperintensity and T1 hypointensity are seen in the periventricular white matter, medial thalamic nuclei, massa intermedia, third ventricular floor, pons, periaqueductal gray matter, and mamillary bodies with enhancement post gadolinium. These changes may reverse after treatment with thiamine.

Submitted by Alan D. S. Chan, MD; Sattam Lingawi, MB, ChB, FRCPC; Peter Brotchie, MBBS, PhD; William G. Bradley, MD, PhD, FACR (Senior Editor), Long Beach Memorial Medical Center, Long Beach, CA.

SUGGESTED READING

Yokote K, Miyagi K, Kuzuhara S, et al. Wernicke's encephalopathy: follow-up study by CT and MR. *JCAT* 1991;15:835–838.

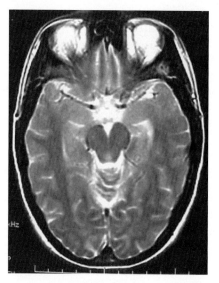

FIGURE 66.1A

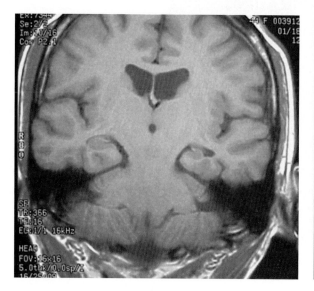

FIGURE 66.1B

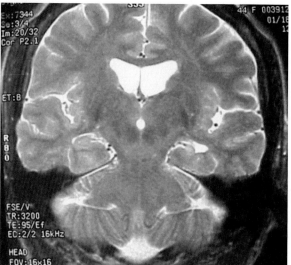

FIGURE 66.1C

CLINICAL HISTORY

A 44-year-old female with epilepsy.

FINDINGS

Axial fast spin-echo T2-weighted image (Fig. 66.1A) demonstrates nonspecific asymmetry in the size of the temporal horns, the left being larger than the right. Thin-section high-resolution coronal T1- and T2-weighted images through the hippocampal formations (Fig. 66.1B,C) demonstrate a small atrophic left hippocampus. Note there is abnormal high signal within the left hippocampus as compared with the right on the T2-weighted acquisition. The left temporal horn is again seen to be larger than the right.

DIAGNOSIS

Left mesial temporal sclerosis (MTS).

DISCUSSION

MTS, also known as hippocampal sclerosis, is the most common cause of medically intractable complex partial seizures, accounting for approximately 65% of cases. Pathologic examination reveals neuronal cell loss, atrophy, and gliosis of the hippocampus. Less commonly, the amygdala or both amygdala and hippocampus are involved. Other mesial temporal structures and/or the entire temporal lobe can be involved. The etiology is not definitely known, although complicated delivery, status epilepticus, and febrile seizures have all been associated with MTS, suggestive of injury of the hippocampus/amygdala at an early age due to hypoxia, hyperpyrexia, or infection.

MRI is the most frequently used imaging modality in the detection of MTS. The most common abnormalities depicted on MRI are unilateral hippocampal atrophy with increased signal intensity on T2-weighted or FLAIR images, reflecting the neuronal cell loss and gliosis. The reported detection rate (or sensitivity) of MRI to hippocampal signal abnormality using T2-weighted acquisition is 93%. The specificity is relatively low (74%). With the addition of secondary signs of MTS such as atrophy of the involved hippocampus and/or temporal lobe, enlargement of the adjacent temporal horn or choroidal fissure, the specificity of MRI is raised to 94% and the diagnosis of hippocampal sclerosis can be more confidently made. Interictal positron emission tomography (PET) scanning can detect temporal lobe hypometabolism on the involved side in 60% to 90% of patients and can confirm cases where MRI has been inconclusive. Other lesions, such as tumor, cavernous angioma, gray matter heterotopia, and stroke, can accompany MTS. It is thought that these lesions are the original epileptogenic foci and that the hippocampal sclerosis is a consequence of the repeated discharges from the adjacent lesion. Occasionally, hippocampal signal abnormality has been identified on MRI without pathologic abnormality. It has been hypothesized that this may be due to seizure activity itself or drug effect.

Surgical resection of the involved temporal lobe offers the best chance at reduction or eradication of seizures in patients with medically intractable temporal lobe epilepsy today. In patients with solitary temporal lobe abnormalities, 86% to 95% of patients will have significant improvement of their seizure disorder following temporal lobectomy.

SUGGESTED READINGS

Heinz R, Ferris N, Lee EK, et al. MR and positron emission tomography in the diagnosis of surgically correctable temporal lobe epilepsy. *AJNR* 1994;15:1341–1348.

Jack CR, Krecke KN, Luetmer PH, et al. Diagnosis of mesial temporal sclerosis with conventional verses fast spin-echo MR imaging. *Radiology* 1994;192:123–127.

Jackson GD, Berkovic SF, Duncan JS, et al. Optimizing the diagnosis of hippocampal sclerosis using MR imaging. *AJNR* 1993;14:753–762.

Lee DH, Gao F, Rogers JM, et al. MR in temporal lobe epilepsy: analysis with pathologic confirmation. *AJNR* 1998;19:19–27.

Meiners LC, van Gils A, Jansen GH, et al. Temporal lobe epilepsy: the various MR appearances of histologically proven mesial temporal sclerosis. *AJNR* 1994;15:1547–1555.

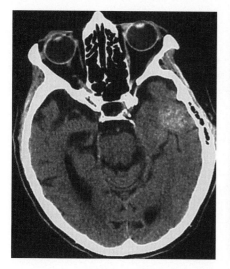

FIGURE 67.1A

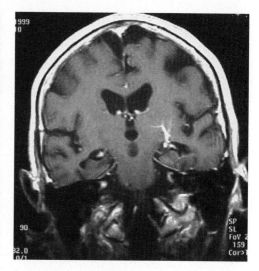

FIGURE 67.1B

FIGURE 67.1C

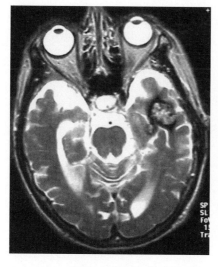

FIGURE 67.1D

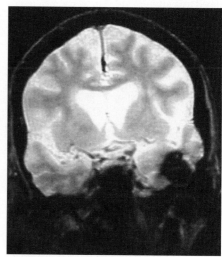

FIGURE 67.1E

CLINICAL HISTORY

An 85-year-old female with mental status change.

FINDINGS

Axial noncontrast computed tomography image (Fig. 67.1A) demonstrates an amorphous rounded collection of high-density material within the left temporal lobe. There is no associated mass effect or edema. Postcontrast T1-weighted acquisitions in the axial and coronal plane (Fig. 67.1B,C) show a 2.5-cm well-defined mass within the left temporal lobe, which is hyperintense centrally with a hypointense rim. Just medial to this lesion is a venous angioma within the left thalamus/temporal lobe. The temporal lobe mass is heterogeneously hyperintense on the T2-weighted acquisition with a complete peripheral rim of low signal consistent with hemosiderin (Fig. 67.1D). Again note lack of perifocal edema or mass effect. Coronal gradient-echo acquisition (Fig. 67.1E) shows significant magnetic susceptibility artifact within the lesion consistent with hemorrhage in varying stages of degradation.

DIAGNOSIS

Cavernous hemangioma with associated venous angioma.

DISCUSSION

The MRI findings of cavernous angioma (Vol. 1, Case 12) and venous angioma (Vol. 1, Case 96) have been discussed elsewhere.

Up to one-third of venous angiomas are associated with cavernous angioma. The simultaneous occurrence of these two entities has been reported to occur more frequently in women and in the posterior fossa. These patients are more likely to experience symptomatic and recurrent hemorrhage. The cavernous angioma is invariably responsible for acute symptomatic hemorrhage and only the cavernoma should be surgically removed. As compared with cavernous angioma alone, cavernoma in association with venous angioma has a lower incidence of seizure and there is less likely to be a history of cavernous angioma in the family.

SUGGESTED READINGS

Abdulrauf SI, Kaynar MY, Awad IA. A comparison of the clinical profile of cavernous malformation with and without associated venous malformation. *Neurosurgery* 1999;44:41–46.

Ostertun B, Solymosi L. Magnetic resonance angiography of cerebral developmental anomalies: its role in differential diagnosis. *Neuroradiology* 1993;35:97–104.

Wilms G, Bleus E, Demaerel P, et al. Simultaneous occurrence of developmental venous anomaly and cavernous angioma. *AJNR* 1994;15:1247–1254.

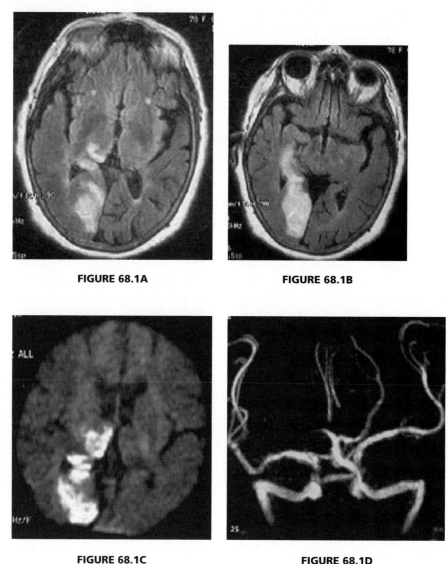

FIGURE 68.1A

FIGURE 68.1B

FIGURE 68.1C

FIGURE 68.1D

CLINICAL HISTORY

A 79-year-old male with sudden onset of left homonymous hemianopsia.

FINDINGS

Axial FLAIR images show increased signal intensity in the right occipital and inferomedial temporal lobes (Fig. 68.1A,B). EPI diffusion sequence shows abnormal increased signal in the same region extending to the right posterior thalamic region (Fig. 68.1C). The MRA shows lack of flow in the distal right posterior cerebral artery (Fig. 68.1D).

DIAGNOSIS

Acute posterior cerebral artery infarction.

DISCUSSION

Diffusion-weighted MRI is a sensitive technique for the early diagnosis of acute cerebral ischemia and infarction. Cerebral ischemia results in cytotoxic edema causing restricted diffusion of water molecules, which results in increased signal on diffusion studies. Infarcts remain hyperintense for 3 weeks. T2-weighted images may show increased signal intensity and mass effect, and enhanced T1-weighted images may show vascular stasis. However, these findings are usually seen after the EPI diffusion image has already become positive.

Several other processes such as tumors, abscesses, and hemorrhage may also result in increased signal intensity on diffusion imaging. Therefore the findings on diffusion imaging should be interpreted in association with other MRI sequence findings and the patient's clinical presentation.

Submitted by Peter Brotchie, MBBS, PhD; Sattam Lingawi, MB, ChB, FRCPC; William G. Bradley, MD, PhD, FACR (Senior Editor), Long Beach Memorial Medical Center, Long Beach, CA.

SUGGESTED READING

Butts K. Isotropic diffusion weighted and spiral navigated EPI for routine imaging of acute stroke. *Magn Reson Med* 1997;38:741–749.

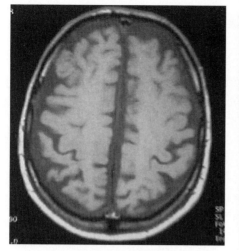

FIGURE 69.1A

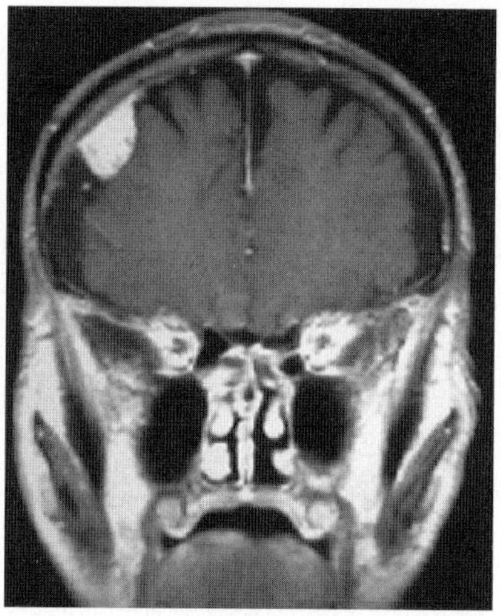

FIGURE 69.1B

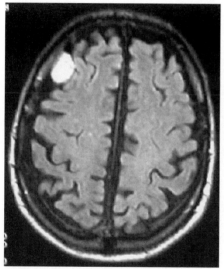

FIGURE 69.1C

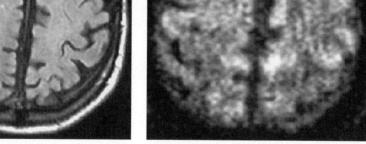

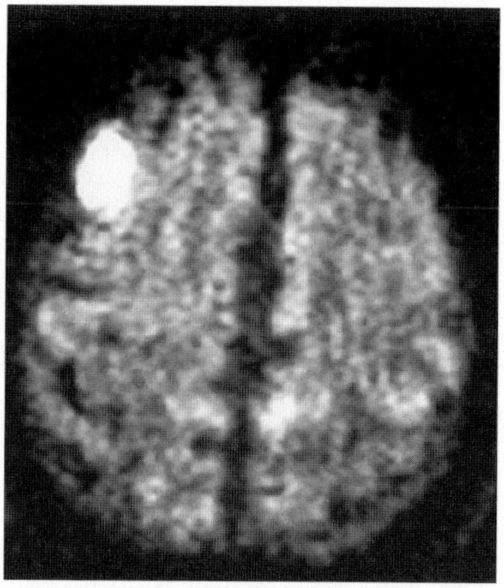

FIGURE 69.1D

CLINICAL HISTORY

An 85-year-old female with a history of headaches and memory loss.

FINDINGS

A 2-cm right frontal extraaxial mass is seen on all images. This is isointense on the axial T1-weighted image (Fig. 69.1A) and shows strong enhancement with a dural tail following administration of gadolinium (Fig. 69.1B). An axial FLAIR image (Fig. 69.1C) and an EPI diffusion image (Fig. 69.1D) show increased signal intensity.

DIAGNOSIS

Right frontal meningioma.

DISCUSSION

Meningiomas tend to be isointense to brain on both T1- and T2-weighted images. The extraaxial location and presence of a dural tail support the diagnosis.

Meningioma is one of the few tumors that can be associated with increased signal on EPI diffusion images along with lymphoma, PNET, and epidermoid. This is due to restricted water motion within the tumor cells (as is also seen in acute infarction). (In the case of lymphoma and PNET, it probably reflects a high nuclear-cytoplasmic ratio, which is the reason these tumors are darker than gliomas on T2-weighted images.)

Meningiomas account for about 15% to 20% of all intracranial malignancies and are of mesodermal origin. They can arise from any of the three meningeal layers. The parasagittal region is the most common site. Dural thickening and enhancement are important aspects of some meningiomas and may be due to meningioepithelial tumor spread or inflammatory changes.

Submitted by Hesham Sabir, MB, ChB; Sattam Lingawi, MB, ChB, FRCPC; Peter Brotchie, MBBS, PhD; William G. Bradley, MD, PhD, FACR (Senior Editor), Long Beach Memorial Medical Center, Long Beach, CA.

SUGGESTED READING

Zee CS. Magnetic resonance imaging of meningiomas. *Semin Ultrasound CT MRI* 1992;13:154–169.

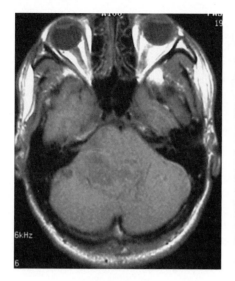

FIGURE 70.1A

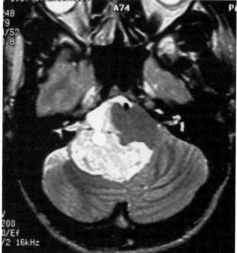

FIGURE 70.1B

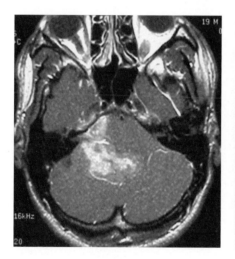

FIGURE 70.1C

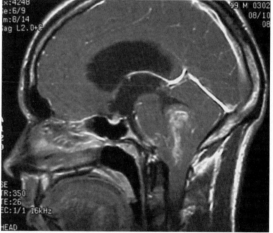

FIGURE 70.1D

CLINICAL HISTORY

A 19-year-old male with morning headaches.

FINDINGS

Axial T1- and T2-weighted images (Fig. 70.1A,B) demonstrate a well-defined heterogeneous mass filling the fourth ventricle with extension into the right cerebellar pontine angle. Axial and sagittal postcontrast T1-weighted acquisitions (Fig. 70.1C,D) demonstrate heterogeneous enhancement. The mass conforms to the configuration of the fourth ventricle and extrudes inferiorly through the foramen magnum. Extension laterally through the right foramen of Luschka into the cerebellar pontine angle is seen again. Note marked enlargement of the lateral and third ventricles consistent with an obstructive hydrocephalus. The tumor does not appear to arise from the brainstem.

DIAGNOSIS

Fourth ventricular ependymoma.

DISCUSSION

Ependymomas account for approximately 10% of all pediatric neoplasms and 5% of all gliomas in all age groups. Ependymomas occur throughout the neuraxis arising from the ependymal lining of the ventricles, central canal, and filum terminale. Intracranial ependymomas are more common in the pediatric age group, whereas spinal tumors occur more frequently in the adult population. Two-thirds of all ependymomas are infratentorial, with the vast majority arising in the fourth ventricle. Most are males with a peak age of 10 to 15 years. Supratentorial tumors are uncommon but can be seen within the brain parenchyma (arising from ectopic ependymal cell rests) or within the lateral ventricle. Supratentorial ependymomas tend to occur in older patients.

Ependymomas are heterogeneous tumors with foci of cystic change, hemorrhage, and calcification. They have the highest frequency of calcification of all posterior fossa tumors. They are known as "plastic or toothpastelike tumors" because of their tendency to form a cast of the ventricle, oozing out the foramen of Luschka and Magendie into the cerebellopontine angle. Tumor often extrudes through the foramen magnum, forming a "tonguelike" projection along the dorsal aspect of the spinal cord (seen in this case). There is usually expansion of the fourth ventricle, with dilatation of its upper aspect forming a "cap" of cerebrospinal fluid (CSF). Ependymomas often invade the floor of the fourth ventricle (pons/medulla) but maintain a distinct cleavage plane between tumor and the cerebellar vermis. The tumor is usually isodense to brain parenchyma on CT. On MRI, the solid portion of the tumor is isointense to gray matter on T1-weighted images, hyperintense on PD-weighted acquisition, and iso- to hyperintense on T2-weighted images. There is mild heterogeneous enhancement following intravenous contrast. Hydrocephalus is invariably present. There is a high incidence of subarachnoid seeding.

Complete surgical resection is difficult, and local recurrence is common. The 5-year survival rate is approximately 50%.

Other differential diagnoses for posterior fossa mass in a child or young adult include medulloblastoma, astrocytoma, and brainstem glioma. Location can help to differentiate these tumors. The medulloblastoma (see Case 40) arises from the superior medullary velum, whereas the astrocytomas (see Case 44) are usually hemispheric. Ependymomas arise anterior to the medullary velum and plexus. Brainstem gliomas arise within the brainstem with posterior displacement of the fourth ventricle as opposed to ventricular expansion (see Case 16).

Ependymomas are the only tumors to extrude through the foramina of the fourth ventricle and are the most heterogeneous tumors to occur in the posterior fossa. Medulloblastomas are classically homogeneous with high density on CT. The degree of enhancement is usually less striking in ependymomas than in medulloblastomas. Astrocytoma is typically a large, cystic mass with enhancing mural nodule. The presence of calcification should favor the diagnosis of ependymoma.

SUGGESTED READINGS

Atlas SW, Ehud Lavi. Intra-axial brain tumors. In: Atlas SW, ed. *Magnetic resonance imaging of the brain and spine*, 2nd ed. Philadelphia: Lippincott-Raven, 1996:378–383.

Lefton DR, Pinto RS, Martin SW. MRI features of intracranial and spinal ependymomas. *Pediatr Neurosurg* 1998;28:97–105.

Spoto GP, Press GA, Hesselink JR, et al. Intracranial ependymoma and subependymoma: MR manifestations. *AJNR* 1990;11:83–91.

Swartz JD, Zimmerman RA, Bilaniuk LT. Computed tomography of intracranial ependymomas. *Radiology* 1982;143:97–101.

Tortori-Donati P, Fondelli, MP, Cama A, et al. Ependymomas of the posterior cranial fossa: CT and MRI findings. *Neuroradiology* 1995;37:238–243.

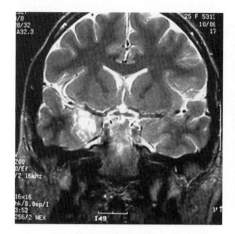

FIGURE 71.1A　　　　　　　　　　　**FIGURE 71.1B**

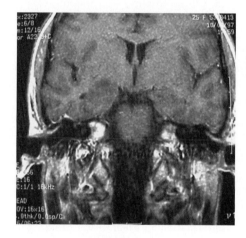　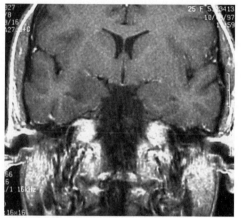

FIGURE 71.1C　　　　　　　　　　　**FIGURE 71.1D**

CLINICAL HISTORY

A 25-year-old female with medically intractable partial complex seizures.

FINDINGS

Targeted T2-weighted images through the hippocampal formations (Fig. 71.1A,B) demonstrate an ill-defined, cortically based multicystic-appearing mass within in the right amygdala. There is perilesional mass effect with mild inferior and lateral displacement of the right hippocampus, best seen in Fig. 71.1B. There is slight superior displacement of the middle cerebral artery on the right. There is no significant perifocal edema. Postcontrast images (Fig. 71.1C,D) show a nonenhancing hypointense mass.

DIAGNOSIS

Dysembryoplastic neuroepithelial (DNET) tumor.

DISCUSSION

DNET is a rare, benign mixed neuroglial tumor. It most commonly presents as chronic partial complex seizures in an adolescent or young adult (typically before the age of 20) without focal neurologic deficit.

On histologic examination, DNET is a benign multinodular lesion composed of glial and neuronal elements. Oligodendrocyte-like cells are mixed with mature ganglion cells and astrocytes in a background of myxoid material. Although DNETs radiographically appear cystic, they are not cystic histopathologically. Dysplastic cortex is often found adjacent to these tumors, leading some to believe that DNETs are actually congenital malformations as opposed to neoplasms.

On CT, DNETs are typically well-defined hypodense masses with marked low-density "cystic" components. Twenty percent of lesions are calcified. Most tumors are supratentorial and intracortical. The most common location is the temporal lobe. Involvement of the caudate nuclei is rare but has been reported. On MRI, the classic description is an intracortical multiloculated "cystic-appearing" mass. DNETs can be multifocal. The tumors are space-occupying lesions and can exhibit mild mass effect. There is usually no peritumoral edema. DNETs are typically hypointense on T1-weighted images (slightly higher signal than CSF), and hyperintense on T2-weighted images. On proton-density acquisition, lesions can be hypo-, iso-, or hyperintense to CSF, reflecting a variable myxoid component. Intralesional hemorrhage has been reported. Solid portions of tumor may enhance. Bony remodeling of the overlying calvarium can be seen, reflecting the early development and indolent nature of DNET.

Surgical resection is the treatment of choice; even with incomplete resection recurrence is uncommon. Radio- and chemotherapy are unwarranted.

Differential diagnosis includes low-grade glioma and ganglioglioma. Gangliogliomas are more often calcified. DNET can mimic a simple cyst; however, tumor signal is usually slightly higher than CSF.

SUGGESTED READINGS

Cervera-Pierot P, Varlet P, Chodkiewicz JP, et al. Dysembryoplastic neuroepithelial tumor located in caudate nucleus area: report of four cases. *Neurosurgery* 1997;40:1065–1069.

Daumas-Duport C, Scheithauer BW, Chodkiewicz JP, et al. Dysembryoplastic neuroepithelial tumor: a surgical curable tumor of young patients with intractable partial seizures. Report of thirty-nine cases. *Neurosurgery* 1988;23:545–556.

Kuroiwa T, Bersey GK, Rothman MI, et al. Radiologic appearance of the dysembryoplastic neuroepithelial tumor. *Radiology* 1995;197:233–238.

Ostertun B, Wolf HK, Campos MG, et al. Dysembryoplastic neuroepithelial tumors: MR and CT evaluation. *AJNR* 1996;17:419–430.

Thom M, Gomez-Anson B, Revesz T, et al. Spontaneous intralesional haemorrhage in dysembryoplastic neuroepithelial tumours: a series of five cases. *J Neurol Neurosurg Psychiatry* 1999;67:97–101.

Whittle IR, Dow GR, Lammie GA, et al. Dysembryoplastic neuroepithelial tumor with discrete bilateral multifocality: further evidence of a germinal origin. *Br J Neurosurg* 1999;13:508–511.

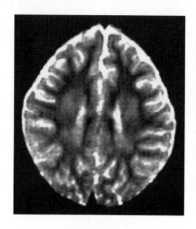

FIGURE 72.1A

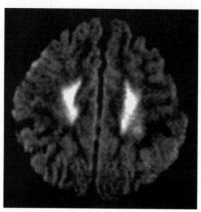

FIGURE 72.1B

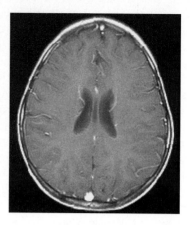

FIGURE 72.1C

CLINICAL HISTORY

A 7-year-old male admitted with drowsiness.

FINDINGS

T2-weighted image shows increased signal in the deep cerebral white matter (Fig. 72.1A). Increased signal is also evident in the white matter on diffusion imaging (Fig. 72.1B). No enhancement is evident with gadolinium (Fig. 72.1C).

DIAGNOSIS

Acute disseminated encephalomyelitis (ADEM).

DISCUSSION

ADEM is a monophasic immune-mediated demyelinating disease that is triggered by a viral infection or a vaccination. On histologic examination, the demyelinating process has a periventricular distribution with infiltration of vascular walls and perivascular space by lymphocytes and plasma cells. Subsequent breakdown of the myelin sheath occurs with preservation of the nerve axonal structure.

The clinical presentation of ADEM is variable and its features are nonspecific. Patients usually present with lethargy, rapid deterioration of consciousness, and convulsions. Other neurologic findings depend on the involved anatomic location.

On T2-weighted MRI, single or multiple high-signal-intensity areas of variable sizes are usually present involving deep and subcortical white matter and that in the basal ganglia. Cortical involvement is rare. These lesions may have mass effect and surrounding edema. Contrast enhancement is variable and is usually in the form of incomplete ring enhancement. These features are nonspecific and could be seen with other forms of encephalitis as well as with multiple sclerosis.

Submitted by Peter Brotchie, MBBS, PhD; Sattam Lingawi, MB, ChB, FRCPC; William G. Bradley, MD, PhD, FACR (Senior Editor), Long Beach Memorial Medical Center, Long Beach, CA.

SUGGESTED READING

Singh S, Alexander M, Korah I. Acute disseminated encephalomyelitis: MR imaging features. *AJR* 1999;173:1101–1107.

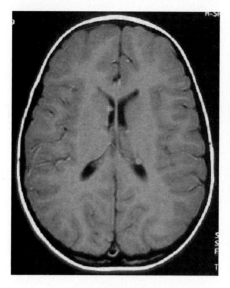

FIGURE 73.1A

FIGURE 73.1B

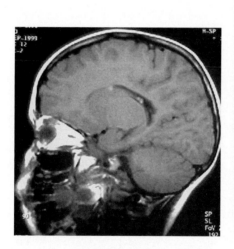

FIGURE 73.1C

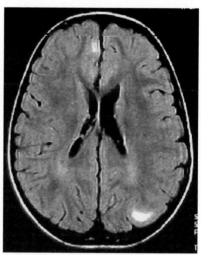

FIGURE 73.1D

CLINICAL HISTORY

A 25-year-old male with facial adenomas and seizures.

FINDINGS

Multiple hyperintense subependymal nodules are evident on the T1-weighted images (Fig. 73.1A,B). These lesions are hypointense on the T2-weighted image (Fig. 73.1C), consistent with calcification. Hyperintense signal abnormalities are evident in the left parietal and right frontal cortex on the T2-weighted and FLAIR images (Fig. 73.1C,D).

DIAGNOSIS

Tuberous sclerosis (TS).

DISCUSSION

TS was first described by von Recklinghausen and later identified as a distinct neurocutaneous syndrome by Bourneville in 1882. It is now recognized as the most frequently occurring neurocutaneous syndrome with the exception of neurofibromatosis type I.

The four major intracranial manifestations of tuberous sclerosis are subependymal nodules, cortical tubers, subependymal giant cell astrocytomas, and white matter radial bands. The latter is thought to represent a migrational disorder where stem cells are arrested at different stages of maturation at different anatomic locations.

On T2-weighted images, enlarged gyri with abnormal configuration and increased signal intensity are often seen, representing cortical tubers (Fig. 73.1C,D). The white matter radial bands are usually seen in the form of high-signal-intensity lines on T2-weighted images extending from the periventricular region to the cortical tubers. These findings are best demonstrated using FLAIR or magnetization transfer (MT) techniques. The subependymal nodules represent hamartomas that may or may not calcify in the teenage years.

The most reliable sign of development of giant cell astrocytoma is a progressive increase in the size of a subependymal nodule. These tend to occur around the foramen of Monro and cause obstructive hydrocephalus. For this reason patients with TS should be followed up with annual MR studies.

Submitted by Sattam Lingawi, MB, ChB; Peter Brotchie, MBBS, PhD; William G. Bradley, MD, PhD, FACR (Senior Editor), Long Beach Memorial Medical Center, Long Beach, CA.

SUGGESTED READING

Seidenwurm DJ, Barkovich AJ. Understanding tuberous sclerosis. *Radiology* 1992;183:23–24.

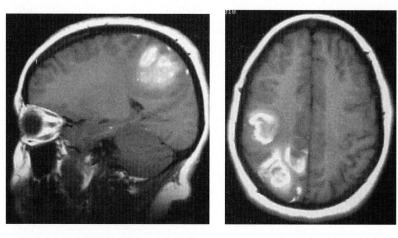

FIGURE 74.1A   **FIGURE 74.1B**

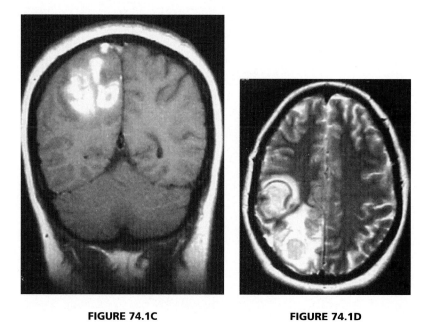

FIGURE 74.1C   **FIGURE 74.1D**

CLINICAL HISTORY

A 37-year-old postpartum female with acute onset of headache and left-sided weakness.

FINDINGS

Sagittal and axial noncontrast T1-weighted acquisition (Fig. 74.1A,B) demonstrate large, multifocal regions of high signal involving the cortex and subcortical white matter of the posterior right parietal lobe. There is surrounding low density consistent with edema. Note the rounded foci of high signal along the surface of the brain consistent with thrombosed cortical veins. On coronal noncontrast T1-weighted acquisition (Fig. 74.1C) there is abnormal high signal within the superior sagittal sinus consistent with thrombosis. Axial T2-weighted images (Fig. 74.1D) demonstrate a heterogeneous signal mass with perifocal edema.

DIAGNOSIS

Superior sagittal sinus thrombosis with hemorrhagic venous infarction.

DISCUSSION

There are several etiologies for focal intraparenchymal hemorrhage, as seen in this case. These include contusion, hypertensive hemorrhage, amyloid angiopathy, venous or arterial infarction, hemorrhagic tumor, vascular malformation, or spontaneous hemorrhage (related to coumadin, amphetamine abuse, or blood dyscrasia).

Venous infarction typically results from occlusion of a major dural venous sinus as well as regional superficial cortical veins. Because of a rich network of venous collateral channels in the brain, if the process is slow (as with meningioma) or limited in extent, no symptoms may be produced. If large venous acute thrombosis occurs, the diminished outflow of blood produces cerebral ischemia and infarction in the underlying brain parenchyma. The territory involved in a venous infarct is quite different from that in arterial infarction. It usually involves the subcortical white matter at the junction between gray and white matter, often appearing as bilateral parasagittal lesions. Hemorrhage is common and typically is identified immediately following the insult, whereas in arterial infarction, hemorrhagic transformation occurs approximately 48 hours after the initial event. There is usually perifocal mass effect. Studies have shown variable T2-weighted signal abnormality in venous infarctions in the absence of hemorrhage. The blood-brain barrier is often not disrupted in venous infarctions; therefore vasogenic edema and enhancement may not be present.

Several different processes can lead to cerebral venous thrombosis (CVT). Local disease processes such as sinusitis/mastoiditis, trauma, and tumor can lead to occlusion of adjacent dural sinuses. Other common associated disorders in adults include (pregnant women, women in the puerperium period and those on oral contraceptives are at increased risk for venous thrombosis) infection, malignancy, collagen vascular diseases, antiphospholipid antibody syndrome, Behçet's disease, and various hematologic diseases. In 25% of cases, no cause is identified. The most common presenting symptom is headache. Additional signs and symptoms include focal sensory or motor neurologic deficit, nausea and vomiting, seizures, and mental status change.

In obstetric CVT, as seen in this case, the diagnosis should be suspected in any woman who develops neurologic symptoms in the immediate postpartum period. CVT occurs more often during puerperium than during pregnancy. Multiparas patients are at slightly increased risk. The postulated mechanism of thrombosis in the obstetric patient is a hypercoagulable state associated with dehydration and anemia. Other factors, such as protein S deficiency, are common during pregnancy, and puerperium may contribute.

Sinus vein thrombosis starts with partial thrombosis of a major dural sinus, most commonly the superior sagittal sinus (SSS). The thrombus progresses to occlude the sinus and then extends into the superficial cortical veins that drain into the SSS (usually anterior to the SSS obstruction). With occlusion of the cortical veins, cortical venous infarctions can occur, frequently with hemorrhagic transformation. After the superior sagittal sinus, the most commonly involved sinuses include the transverse, sigmoid, and cavernous sinuses in descending order of frequency. The internal cerebral veins are less commonly involved but result in severe neurologic sequelae. With extension of clot into the vein of Galen and straight sinus, infarction of the basal ganglia, upper midbrain, thalami, and adjacent white matter can result.

The classic finding of CVT on noncontrast CT is hyperdense material within, and expansion of, the involved dural sinus. Thrombosed cortical veins may be seen as linear high-density regions (cord sign). With contrast, there is enhancement of the meningeal veins and collateral venous channels that surround the relatively low-density venous clot, creating the "empty delta sign."

On MRI, signal abnormality varies with clot age. Clot is most commonly seen in the subacute phase and is hyperintense on T1- and T2-weighted images. Acute thrombosis can be difficult to detect, as it is typically isointense on T1-weighted images and hypointense on T2-weighted acquisition, simulating flow-void. Chronic thrombosis can also be elusive, as hemosiderin is hypointense (similar to flowing blood) on both T1- and T2-weighted images. Gradient-echo images can be helpful in the diagnosis. The normal hyperintense flow seen in patent dural sinuses is replaced by signal void when clot is present.

Two-dimensional (2D) time-of-flight (TOF) MR angiography (MRA) and 2D phase contrast (PC) imaging are useful modalities in assessing intracranial venous flow because of their sensitivity to slow flow. Sagittal 2D PC and coronal 2D TOF MRA are best for evaluating the SSS. Coronal 2D TOF imaging is optimal because flow-related enhancement is optimal when flow into the imaging plane is perpendicular to the imaging slice. Signal is lost when vessels are parallel to the imaging plane (creating signal loss in the posterior aspect of the SSS on coronal 2D TOF images). Another common pitfall is the misinterpretation of hyperintense clot (methemoglobin) as high signal flow on 2D TOF images. Correlation should always be made with T1-weighted SE images to avoid this mistake. 2D PC is a useful technique because of its sensitivity to flow in all directions. The complex flow within the torcula and sigmoid sinuses is better evaluated than with 2D PC MR venography. PC techniques are sensitive to flow only and will not incorporate high signal on T1-weighted images (methemoglobin) into the image as seen with 2D TOF technique. The disadvantage of PC techniques is the acquisition and postprocessing manipulation required and the difficulty in identifying nonobstructive, intraluminal thrombus.

SUGGESTED READINGS

Applegate GR, Talagala SL, Apple LJ. MR angiography of the head and neck: value of two-dimensional phase-contrast projection technique. *AJR* 1992;159:369–374.

Bakshi R, Lindsay BD, Bates VE, et al. Cerebral venous infarctions presenting as enhancing space occupying lesions: MRI findings. *J Neuroimaging* 1998;8:210–215.

Johnson BA, Fram EK. Cerebral venous occlusive disease: pathophysiology, clinical manifestations, and imaging. *Neuroimag Clin North Am* 1992;2:769–783.

Lavin PJM, Bone I, Lamb JT, et al. Intracranial venous thrombosis in the first trimester of pregnancy. *J Neurol Neurosurg* 1978;41:726–729.

Mattle HP, Wentz KU, Edelman RR, et al. Cerebral venography with MR. *Radiology* 1991;178:453–458.

Padayachee TS, Bingham JB, Graves MF, et al. Dural sinus thrombosis: diagnosis and follow-up by magnetic resonance angiography and imaging. *Neuroradiology* 1991;33:165–167.

Perl J II, Turski PA, Masaryk TJ. MR angiography. Techniques and clinical applications. In: Atlas SW, ed. *Magnetic resonance imaging of the brain and spine*, 2nd ed. Philadelphia: Lippincott-Raven 1996:1586–1589.

Yuh WT, Simonson TM, Wang AM, et al. Venous sinus occlusive disease: MR findings. *AJNR* 1994;15:309–316.

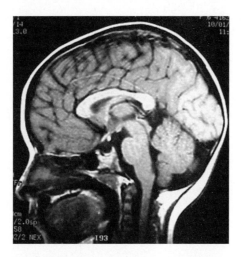

FIGURE 75.1A

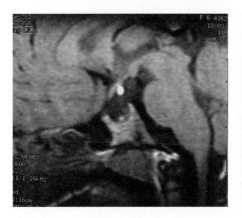

FIGURE 75.1B

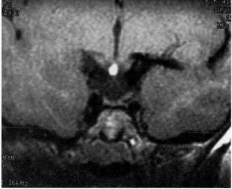

FIGURE 75.1C

CLINICAL HISTORY

A 6-year-old female presents with growth retardation.

FINDINGS

Sagittal T1-weighted acquisition (Fig. 75.1A) shows absence of the normal infundibulum. There is a partially empty sella turcica. The normal posterior pituitary bright spot is not identified within the sella turcica. There is an abnormal focus of high signal immediately posterior to the optic chiasm along the inferior aspect of the hypothalamus. Findings are confirmed on thin-section, targeted images through the sella turcica in the sagittal and coronal plane (Fig. 75.1B,C).

DIAGNOSIS

Ectopic posterior pituitary gland.

DISCUSSION

Approximately 10% of patients with short stature and growth retardation have congenital pituitary dwarfism, which is caused by an idiopathic deficiency of growth hormone. Many of these patients also exhibit deficiencies in anterior pituitary hormones. With the advent of MRI, complex neurohypophyseal abnormalities can be better identified; a constellation of characteristic imaging features has been described in many of these patients. The MRI findings consist of one or more of the following: severe hypoplasia or absence of the infundibulum, absent posterior pituitary "bright spot" within the sella turcica, small (3- to 8-mm) nodule of high signal on T1-weighted images along the median eminence immediately posterior to the optic chiasm (ectopic posterior pituitary gland), and a small anterior pituitary gland with or without hypoplastic sella turcica. More than 40% of patients with idiopathic growth hormone deficiency have been reported to have an ectopic neurohypophysis with associated absent or hypoplastic infundibulum.

The etiology of this anomaly is uncertain. One of the proposed hypotheses is a perinatal ischemic event related to trauma because of the high incidence of breech delivery in these patients. Another theory is congenital maldevelopment of the midline structures with failure of the neurohypophysis to descend completely into the sella turcica. Associated midline anomalies seen at imaging in the pituitary dwarf include absent septum pellucidum and optic nerve hypoplasia. Proponents of this theory suggest that the resultant abnormal fetal pituitary gland function affects fetal position and delivery, accounting for the high incidence of breech delivery in these patients.

The high signal within the ectopic posterior pituitary gland on T1-weighted acquisition is thought to be due to lipid material within the cytoplasm of the normal pituicytes. It has also been postulated that the hyperintense T1-weighted signal is related to the inherent short T1 characteristics of the neurohypophyseal neurosecretory material (ADH/neurophysin complex).

The primary functional abnormality in these patients is thought to be the absent or hypoplastic infundibulum. This results in decreased blood flow to the anterior pituitary lobe with variable degrees of hypopituitarism. The continued axonal neurosecretion at the median eminence, however, stimulates proliferation of rest cell pituicytes, resulting in regeneration of the posterior pituitary gland in an ectopic location. The ectopic gland secretes ADH as a normally located neurohypophysis would; therefore diabetes insipidus is not present in these patients.

An "ectopic pituitary bright spot" has also been reported in patients with sellar or parasellar tumors. In these cases, the ectopic gland regenerates in an ectopic location as a result of the tumor compressing and/or destroying the posterior lobe of the gland or following hypophysectomy.

The possibility that the suprasellar "bright spot" represents a fatty tumor such as lipoma or dermoid can be excluded by the fact that an ectopic posterior pituitary gland will demonstrate increased signal relative to subcutaneous fat or marrow on proton-density and T2-weighted images.

SUGGESTED READINGS

Abrahams JJ, Trefelner E, Boulware SD. Idiopathic growth hormone deficiency: MR findings in 35 patients. *AJNR* 1991;12:155–160.

El Gammal T, Brooks BS, Hoffman WH. MR imaging of the ectopic bright signal of posterior pituitary regeneration. *AJNR* 1989;10:323–328.

Fahrendorf G, Branswig J, Bals-Pratsch M. MR findings in patients with idiopathic panhypopituitarism. *Rofo Fortschr Geb Rontgenstr Neuen Bildgeb Verfahr* 1990;552:550–555.

Hamilton J, Blaser S, Daneman D. MR imaging in idiopathic growth hormone deficiency. *AJNR* 1998;19:1609–1615.

Kelly WM, Kucharczyk W, Kucharczyk J, et al. Posterior pituitary ectopia: an MR feature of pituitary dwarfism. *AJNR* 1988;9:453–460.

Ochi M, Morikawa M, Yoshimoto M, et al. Growth retardation due to idiopathic growth hormone deficiencies: MR findings in 24 patients. *Pediatr Radiol* 1992;22:477–480.

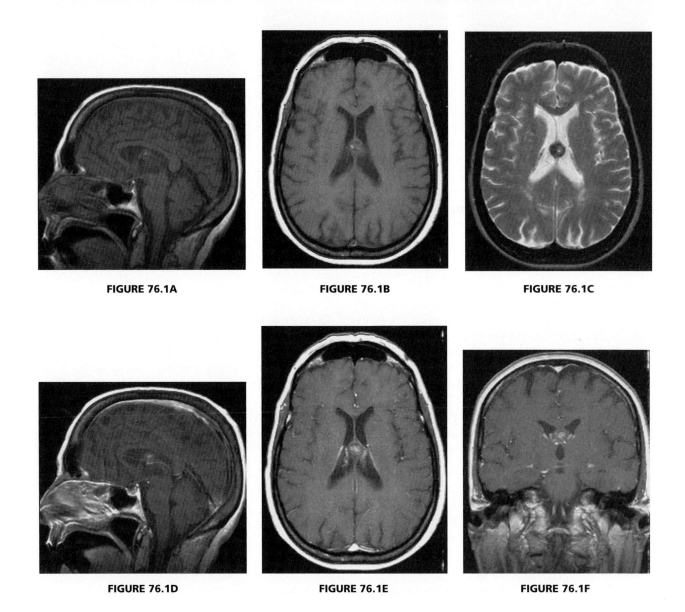

FIGURE 76.1A　　　　**FIGURE 76.1B**　　　　**FIGURE 76.1C**

FIGURE 76.1D　　　　**FIGURE 76.1E**　　　　**FIGURE 76.1F**

CLINICAL HISTORY

A 78-year-old female presenting with headaches.

FINDINGS

A 12-mm round, heterogeneous, intraventricular mass is located in the midline superior to the third ventricle, arising from the septum pellucidum (Fig. 76.1A–C). This demonstrates mild mass effect on the medial aspect of the lateral ventricles bilaterally, but there is no evidence for hydrocephalus or midline shift. There are areas of dark signal on the T2-weighted sequence compatible with either calcification or flow voids (Fig. 76.1C), as well as mild heterogeneous enhancement on the postcontrast images (Fig. 76.1D–F).

DIAGNOSIS

Central neurocytoma.

DISCUSSION

Central neurocytomas are rare, benign masses, constituting approximately 0.5% of primary brain tumors. They are intraventricular and are usually found adjacent to the foramen of Monro or septum pellucidum. They are well-defined, sharply circumscribed, lobulated, vascular tumors that can demonstrate areas of necrosis and uncommonly lead to frank intraventricular hemorrhage. They are indistinguishable from oligodendrogliomas by light microscopy, and in the past have been referred to as *intraventricular oligodendrogliomas*. Their neuronal origin is confirmed by electron microscopy findings, in which they are found to contain neurosecretory granules, synapses, microtubules, and neuritic processes. On immunohistochemical studies, they are found to express neuronal marker proteins, neuron-specific enolase, and synaptophysin.

The common clinical presentation is an adult patient complaining of several months of headaches and signs of increased intracranial pressure. The average age of presentation is 31 years, with a range of 17 to 53 years. Survival has been seen for up to 19 years, and no deaths have been reported from tumor growth or recurrent neoplasm.

By MRI, central neurocytomas are characteristically inhomogeneously isointense on T1-weighted images and demonstrate variable signal characteristics on T2-weighted images with areas of decreased signal representing calcification or tumor vessels. Enhancement patterns are inhomogeneous and range from absent to moderate. By CT, these masses are iso- or slightly hyperdense, and demonstrate a broad-based attachment to the superolateral ventricular wall. They may contain multiple small cysts or clumped, coarse, or globular calcifications and typically demonstrate mild to moderate contrast enhancement. Hydrocephalus is often present. Most central neurocytomas are avascular by angiography; however, some demonstrate moderate to marked vascularity.

The differential diagnosis should include oligodendrogliomas, subependymal giant cell astrocytoma, low-grade or pilocytic astrocytoma, and ependymoma.

Submitted by Elizabeth Vogler, MD; Peter Brotchie, MBBS, PhD; William G. Bradley, MD, PhD, FACR (Senior Editor), Long Beach Memorial Medical Center, Long Beach, CA.

SUGGESTED READING

Osborn AG. *Diagnostic neuroradiology*. St. Louis: Mosby, 1994;582–584.

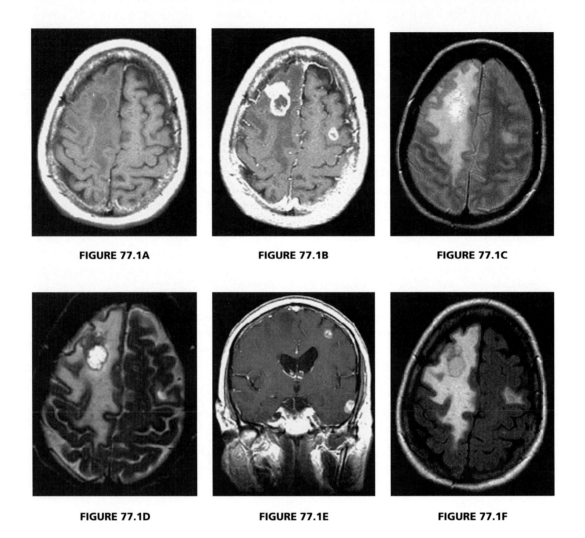

FIGURE 77.1A   **FIGURE 77.1B**   **FIGURE 77.1C**

FIGURE 77.1D   **FIGURE 77.1E**   **FIGURE 77.1F**

CLINICAL HISTORY

An elderly male with lung cancer.

FINDINGS

Multiple ring-enhancing lesions are present in both cerebral hemispheres, primarily at the gray-white junction (Fig. 77.1A–F). These lesions range in size from a few millimeters to approximately 1 cm. A significant amount of associated vasogenic edema surrounds the masses (Fig. 77.1C,D,F). No hemorrhage or ischemia is identified.

DIAGNOSIS

Parenchymal metastases.

DISCUSSION

Metastatic disease to the brain usually occurs via the hematogenous route. The most common manifestation is parenchymal involvement followed by disease affecting the skull, leptomeninges, and dura. Rarely, carcinomatous encephalitis or paraneoplastic disease can occur.

Metastatic disease usually involves older adults and can be clinically silent, or it can result in neurologic symptoms, which depend on the areas of involvement. It accounts for approximately a quarter to a third of all tumors affecting the brain.

Common primary extracranial tumors that metastasize to the brain parenchyma include lung, breast, melanoma, and less commonly gastrointestinal and genitourinary tumors. Metastatic deposits are typically well circumscribed, multiple, and variable in size. The most common parenchymal location is within the white matter, especially at the corticomedullary junctions. There is commonly a disproportionate amount of surrounding vasogenic edema relative to the size of the mass. On nonenhanced CT (NECT), the vasogenic edema may be the only finding. The lesions are usually isodense on NECT. Hyperdense metastases are usually seen with small round cell tumors or tumors with high nuclear-to-cytoplasmic ratios. Hemorrhage can be seen with certain tumors such as renal, breast, thyroid, lung, melanoma, or choriocarcinoma. There is usually intense enhancement in either a solid or ring-enhancing pattern.

Metastatic disease is usually slightly hypointense to normal brain parenchyma on T1 and hyperintense on T2. In contrast, metastatic melanoma may exhibit high T1 signal intensities, depending on the melanin content and presence of subacute hemorrhage. Some metastatic tumors such as mucin-secreting tumors or highly cellular tumors demonstrate low T2 signal intensities on T2-weighted images. Hemorrhage also complicates the typical signal intensity pattern. Contrast-enhanced MR is the most sensitive. The enhancement pattern may be solid, rim, or heterogeneous.

Differential considerations include multifocal primary tumors or infection.

Submitted by Stephanie Y. Chiu, MD; Sattam Lingawi MB, ChB, FRCPC; Peter Brotchie, MBBS, PhD; William G. Bradley, MD, PhD, FACR (Senior Editor), Long Beach Memorial Medical Center, Long Beach, CA.

SUGGESTED READING

Osborn, AG. *Diagnostic neuroradiology*. St. Louis: Mosby, 1994:657–668.

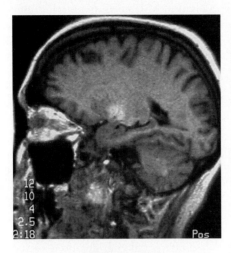

FIGURE 78.1A

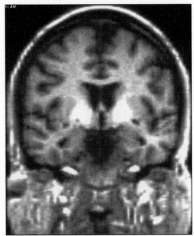

FIGURE 78.1B

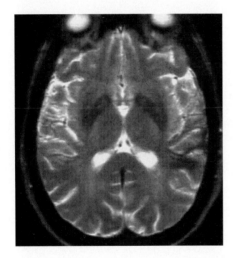

FIGURE 78.1C

CLINICAL HISTORY

A 47-year-old alcoholic female with liver disease.

FINDINGS

Sagittal and coronal noncontrast T1-weighted acquisition (Fig. 78.1A,B) demonstrates abnormal, poorly defined hyperintense signal within the basal ganglia bilaterally. No signal abnormality is identified in this region of the T2-weighted image (Fig. 78.1C).

DIAGNOSIS

Metabolic alteration of basal ganglia related to chronic liver disease.

DISCUSSION

The relationship of high-signal abnormalities in the basal ganglia with chronic liver disease was recognized in the late 1980s. In many such patients, large portal/systemic collateral vessels were documented. Such lesions do not always correlate with neurologic symptoms or change in mental status, although portal-systemic encephalopathy is often associated with the findings. High signal intensity in the basal ganglia can be seen with elevation of lipid content, hemorrhagic byproducts (such as methemoglobin) and even floccular calcification. Manganese shows a paramagnetic effect and appears to have a preferential affinity for the globus pallidus. This could also produce the abnormality.

It is generally believed that gut-derived toxins that normally do not have access to the brain are responsible for the eventual production of high signal intensity in the basal ganglia whether it is on the basis of trace metal accumulation or that of some other factors not yet established.

SUGGESTED READINGS

Brunberg JA, Kanal E, Hirsch W, et al. Chronic acquired hepatic failure: MR imaging of the brain at 1.5 T. *AJNR* 1991;12:909–914.

Mirowitz SA, Westrich TJ, Hirsch JD. Hyperintense basal ganglia on T1-weighted MR images in patients receiving parenteral nutrition. *Radiology* 1991;181:117–120.

Zeneroli ML, Cioni G, Crisi G, et al. Globus pallidus alterations and brain atrophy in liver cirrhosis patients with encephalopathy: an MR imaging study. *Magn Reson Imaging* 1991;9:295–302.

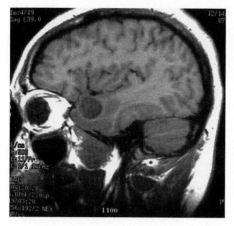

FIGURE 79.1A

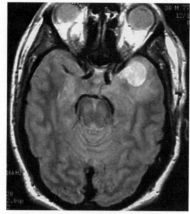

FIGURE 79.1B

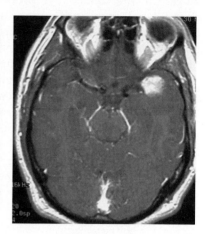

FIGURE 79.1C

CLINICAL HISTORY

A 39-year-old male with a history of medically intractable partial complex seizures.

FINDINGS

Noncontrast sagittal T1-weighted acquisition (Fig. 79.1A) demonstrates a well-defined hypointense mass involving the cortex and subcortical white matter of the anterior medial aspect of the left temporal lobe. The lesion is well defined and hyperintense on the proton-density acquisition (Fig. 79.1B). Note minimal peritumoral edema. Following intravenous contrast (Fig. 79.1C), there is intense, homogeneous enhancement.

DIAGNOSIS

Ganglioglioma.

DISCUSSION

Gangliogliomas are rare primary central nervous system tumors composed of both dysplastic neuronal and astrocytic elements, which can be found throughout the neuraxis but are most commonly located within the temporal lobe. They typically occur in children and young adults. Sixty percent to 80 percent of patients are under 30 years of age. Seizures are the most common presenting complaint. Focal neurologic deficits and signs of increased intracranial pressure can occur. The tumor is very slow growing and symptoms are usually long-standing (mean of 11 years before diagnosis).

Tumors can be solid or cystic. They are typically hypodense on CT. The lesions are hypointense on T1-weighted images and hyperintense on T2-weighted images. There is typically little to no perifocal edema. Calcification occurs in approximately 50% of cases. Enhancement is variable, ranging from none to striking. Enhancement pattern can be nodular, rim, and/or solid. There can be remodeling or scalloping of the overlying bony calvarium in superficial lesions. A commonly described imaging appearance is that of a cystic lesion with partially calcified mural nodule. This presentation, however, only occurs in 50% of cases.

Most gangliogliomas are low-grade tumors with a favorable prognosis. Higher-grade tumors can occur when there is anaplasia of the astrocytic component. Significant peritumoral edema on CT or MRI is suggestive of higher-grade ganglioglioma. Fluorodeoxyglucose-positron emission tomography (FDG-PET) and thallium 201-SPECT scanning can also be helpful in identifying higher-grade tumors preoperatively. Metastasis is rare but has been reported to the leptomeninges and subarachnoid space.

Total surgical resection is the treatment of choice. Even with subtotal resection, the prognosis is good for not only survival but seizure control. There is currently no role for postoperative radiation treatment or chemotherapy.

The main differential diagnosis for a cystic ganglioglioma is juvenile pilocytic astrocytoma and pleomorphic xanthoastrocytoma, both of which typically present as a cystic mass with mural nodule. The ganglioglioma is the most likely tumor of the three to calcify.

SUGGESTED READINGS

Castillo M. Ganglioglioma: ubiquitous or not? *AJNR* 1998;19:807–809.

Kincaid DK, el-Saden SM, Park SH, et al. Cerebral ganglioglioma: preoperative grading using FDG-PET and 201 Tl-SPECT. *AJNR* 1998;19:801–806.

Matsumoto K, Tamiya T, Ono Y, et al. Cerebral ganglioglioma: clinical characteristics, CT and MRI. *Acta Neurochir (Wien)* 1999;141:135–140.

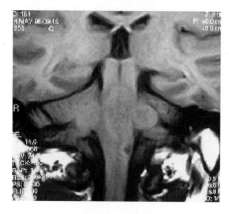

FIGURE 80.1A

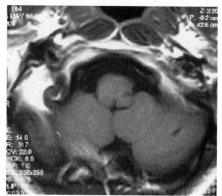

FIGURE 80.1B

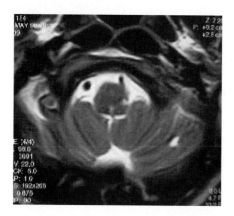

FIGURE 80.1C

CLINICAL HISTORY

A 51-year-old female with sudden onset of left facial and right body numbness.

FINDINGS

Low T1 and high T2 signal is evident within a well-defined focus on the left side of the medulla (Fig. 80.1A–C).

DIAGNOSIS

Lateral medullary infarct.

DISCUSSION

Small infarctions of the lateral medulla produce a typical constellation of neurologic deficit that can be fairly reliably recognized clinically.

A full-blown Wallenberg's syndrome consists of contralateral loss numbness in the body (spinothalamic tract), ipsilateral numbness in the face (trigeminal spinal tract), Horner's syndrome (descending sympathetics), trouble swallowing and hoarseness (nucleus ambiguous), and hemiparesis (corticospinal tract).

Although CT often fails to visualize medullary infarcts due to beam-hardening artifacts, MRI successfully demonstrates even very small medullary infarcts. However, identification of small infarcts can be difficult if the slice thickness is too large. Thin sections result in lower signal to noise, which can be improved with signal averaging at the expense of increased scan time.

Like other brain infarcts, medullary infarcts have low signal on T1- and high signal on T2-weighted images. Diffusion imaging is the most sensitive modality for early detection of medullary infarcts. MRI is also useful in the evaluation of the vertebral arteries for evidence of vascular occlusion, which is recognized by a loss of the normal flow void. MR angiography is often helpful in these situations.

Submitted by Sattam Lingawi, MB, ChB; Peter Brotchie, MBBS, PhD; William G. Bradley, MD, PhD, FACR (Senior Editor), Long Beach Memorial Medical Center, Long Beach, CA.

SUGGESTED READING

Fox AJ, Bogousslavsky J, Carey LS, et al. Magnetic resonance imaging of small medullary infarction. *AJNR* 1986;7:229–233.

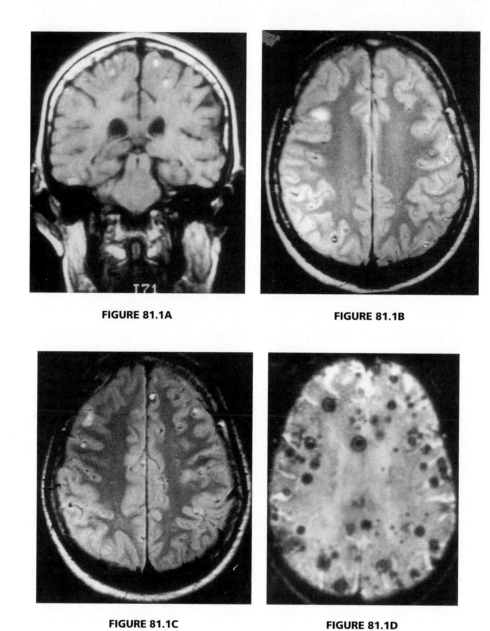

FIGURE 81.1A

FIGURE 81.1B

FIGURE 81.1C

FIGURE 81.1D

CLINICAL HISTORY

A 56-year-old female with headaches.

FINDINGS

T1-weighted (Fig. 81.1A), proton-density-weighted (Fig. 81.1B), and T2-weighted (Fig. 81.1C) images demonstrate scattered punctate areas of high signal with surrounding low-intensity rims. A low flip angle, T2-weighted gradient-echo image (Fig. 81.1D) demonstrates multiple areas of low signal intensity.

DIAGNOSIS

Hemorrhagic metastases.

DISCUSSION

Conventional spin-echo imaging in this case demonstrates punctate areas of hemorrhage that are bright on both T1- and T2-weighted images with a low-intensity rim, best seen on the T2-weighted images. These findings are consistent with extracellular methemoglobin surrounded by a hemosiderin rim (i.e., chronic hemorrhage). The number of lesions detected with the low-flip-angle, T2-weighted gradient-echo image, however, is much greater. This indicates the great sensitivity of gradient-echo images for detecting magnetically susceptible forms of hemorrhage, that is, acute hemorrhage (intracellular deoxyhemoglobin), early subacute hemorrhage (intracellular methemoglobin), and chronic hemorrhage (hemosiderin rim). In general, the sensitivity to susceptibility effects such as these increases with increasing field strength, gradient-echo technique (as opposed to spin echo or fast spin echo), and T2-weighting (long TE and low flip angle).

The metastases, which are commonly hemorrhagic, include bronchogenic (as in this case), melanoma, renal cell, thyroid, choriocarcinoma, and breast. Ten percent to 30% of patients with MR-detectable metastatic disease will have a normal neurologic examination.

Submitted by William G. Bradley, MD, PhD, FACR (Senior Editor), Long Beach Memorial Medical Center, Long Beach, CA.

SUGGESTED READING

Bradley WG. Hemorrhage. In: Stark DD, Bradley WG, eds. *Magnetic resonance imaging*, 3rd ed. St. Louis: Mosby, 1999:1329–1346.

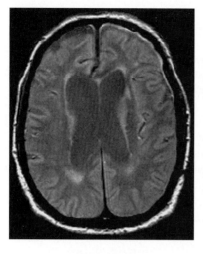

FIGURE 82.1A

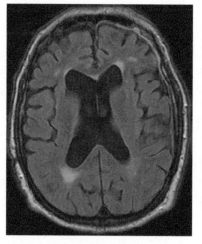

FIGURE 82.1B

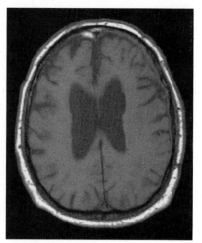

FIGURE 82.1C

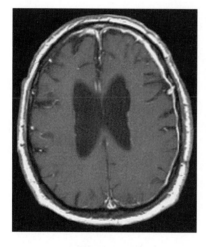

FIGURE 82.1D

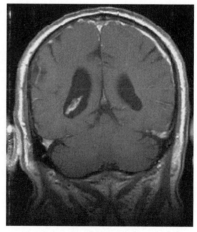

FIGURE 82.1E

CLINICAL HISTORY

A 67-year-old female with history of dementia, repeated falls, and head injuries.

FINDINGS

Thin, hyperintense, extraaxial collection is evident over the surface of the left frontal lobe on the proton-density and FLAIR images (Fig. 82.1A,B). The collection is low signal on T1-weighted images with marked enhancement following administration of gadolinium.

DIAGNOSIS

Chronic subdural hematoma.

DISCUSSION

The blood products in a subdural hematoma evolve through similar stages to blood within an intraparenchymal hemorrhage, but at a slower rate. Subdural collections are recognized by their distinctive concave shape.

The appearance of blood products on MRI depends on several factors, especially the specific form of hemoglobin. Initially, oxygen is bound to hemoglobin (oxyhemoglobin) and is diamagnetic (i.e., no unpaired electrons). It causes neither T1 nor T2 shortening and is isointense on T1- and hyperintense on T2-weighted ("hyperacute" state) images.

When the hemoglobin becomes deoxygenated (deoxyhemoglobin), it is paramagnetic (with four unpaired electrons), causing T2 shortening. Deoxyhemoglobin appears hypointense on both T1- and T2-weighted images ("acute" hemorrhage).

With time the deoxyhemoglobin is oxidized to methemoglobin, which is also paramagnetic (with five unpaired electrons). Early subacute hemorrhage (intact red blood cells) has high T1 and low T2 signal, whereas late subacute hemorrhage (lysed red blood cells) is hyperintense on both T1- and T2-weighted images.

In chronic subdural hematomas the signal is somewhat greater than that of cerebrospinal fluid (CSF) on T1- and T2-weighted images, reflecting the higher protein content. If the collection becomes vascularized, enhancement will be seen with gadolinium.

Submitted by Peter Brotchie, MBBS, PhD; Sattam Lingawi, MB, ChB, FRCPC; William G. Bradley, MD, PhD, FACR (Senior Editor), Long Beach Memorial Medical Center, Long Beach, CA.

SUGGESTED READING

Gomori JM, Grossman RI. Mechanisms responsible for the MRI appearance and evolution of intracranial hemorrhage. *Radiographics* 1988;8:427–440.

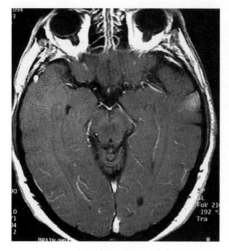

FIGURE 83.1A

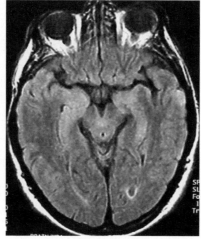

FIGURE 83.1B

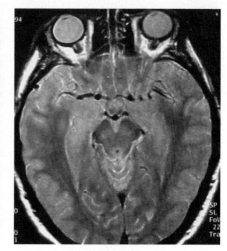

FIGURE 83.1C

CLINICAL HISTORY

A 67-year-old male with auditory hallucinations and aphasia.

FINDINGS

Axial postcontrast T1-weighted acquisition (Fig. 83.1A) demonstrates enhancement of a single gyrus within the left temporal lobe. No other focal regions of intracranial enhancement are identified. On the axial FLAIR acquisition (Fig. 83.1B) there is very subtle hyperintense signal in this region. No signal abnormality could be identified on the proton-density or T2-weighted image (Fig. 83.1C).

DIAGNOSIS

Gyral infarct.

DISCUSSION

In rare cases, MRI scanning will be negative in the subacute phase of a small infarct, and only the abnormal blood-brain barrier as depicted by contrast-enhanced scanning will provide the diagnosis. Diffusion sequences typically will be helpful in the first 2 weeks, demonstrating the acute nature of ischemia, but starting a week after the event these may also be falsely negative for a subacute infarct. The gyral nature of the enhancement indicating predominantly gray matter involvement and a history of acute onset of the event lead to the correct diagnosis.

SUGGESTED READINGS

Baron JC, von Kummer R, Del Zoppo GJ. Treatment of acute ischemic stroke: challenging the concept of a rigid and universal time window. *Stroke* 1995;26:2219–2221.

Russell EJ. Diagnosis of hyperacute ischemic infarct with CT: key to improved clinical outcome after intravenous thrombolysis? *Radiology* 1997;205:315–318.

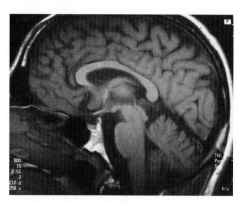

FIGURE 84.1A

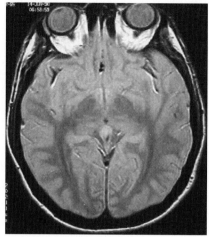

FIGURE 84.1B

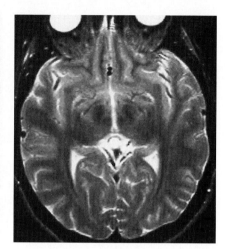

FIGURE 84.1C

CLINICAL HISTORY

A 25-year-old male presents with headache.

FINDINGS

Sagittal T1-weighted acquisition (Fig. 84.1A) demonstrates a region of intermediate signal in the expected location of the pineal gland immediately posterior to the superior colliculi. Axial proton-density and T2-weighted images (Fig. 84.1B,C) demonstrate a less than 1-cm, rounded, well-defined mass that is isointense to cerebral spinal fluid on both pulse sequences. There is no perifocal mass effect. The ventricles are normal in size.

DIAGNOSIS

Pineal cyst.

DISCUSSION

Pineal cysts are nonneoplastic benign cystic lesions that are lined by collagenous fibers, glial cells, and normal pineal parenchymal cells. Small pineal cysts are common incidental findings and have been found in up to 40% of autopsy series. The prevalence of pineal cysts on MRI (typically defined as greater than 5 mm) has been reported in up to 10% of individuals in different studies. Their cause is uncertain. Theories include degenerative change, coalescence of smaller cysts, sequestration of the pineal diverticulum, and/or failure of normal pineal gland development. Most pineal cysts are found in young women (21 to 30 years of age). The incidence seems to decrease with age. Most cases are asymptomatic. Even large lesions with local mass effect (i.e., compression of the cerebral aqueduct or tectal plate) are usually without associated symptoms. Occasionally, pineal cysts can hemorrhage acutely and compress the cerebral aqueduct, resulting in hydrocephalus and Parinaud's syndrome. There is a greater incidence of symptomatic pineal cysts in women.

Pineal cysts can be difficult to distinguish from small cystic neoplasms. The MR diagnosis is based mainly on morphology as opposed to signal characteristics. The pineal cyst is round, with smooth margins. It can lie within a portion of the gland or replace the entire structure. The signal characteristics of the cyst fluid on MRI follows cerebrospinal fluid (CSF) on all pulse sequences or may have a slightly higher signal than CSF (best seen on FLAIR or proton-density images). This is probably related to higher protein content, old hemorrhage, and/or isolation from CSF flow effect. A pineal cyst should not enhance centrally. Peripheral enhancement can be seen due to enhancement of normal surrounding pineal tissue, which usually lacks a blood-brain barrier. The presence of tumor heterogeneity (related to calcification, hemorrhage, fat, or soft tissue), central enhancement, and/or parapineal site of origin should raise suspicion for neoplasm. Gradient-echo imaging is useful in the detection of small foci of calcification and/or hemorrhage. Clinical history and follow-up imaging to ascertain lesion stability can also be helpful in distinguishing pineal cyst from cystic neoplasm. Significant improvement in microsurgical technique in recent years has made biopsy and/or cyst aspiration an option in difficult cases.

SUGGESTED READINGS

Golzarian J, Baleriaux D, Bank WO, et al. Pineal cyst: normal or pathologic? *Neuroradiology* 1993;35:251–253.

Jinkins JR, Xiong L, Reiter RJ. The midline pineal "eye": MR and CT characteristics of the pineal gland with and without benign cyst formation. *J Pineal Res* 1995;19:64–71.

Miyatake S, Kikuchi H, Yamasaki T, et al. Glial cyst of the pineal gland with characteristic computed tomography, magnetic resonance imaging, and pathological findings: report of 2 cases. *Surg Neurol* 1992;37:293–299.

Sawamura Y, Ikeda J, Ozawa M, et al. MRI reveals a high incidence of asymptomatic pineal cysts in young females. *J Neurosurg* 1995;37:11–15.

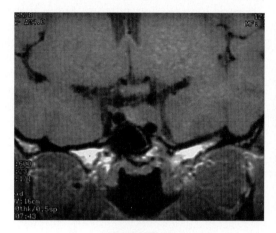

FIGURE 85.1A

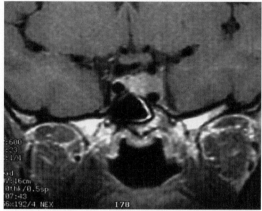

FIGURE 85.1B

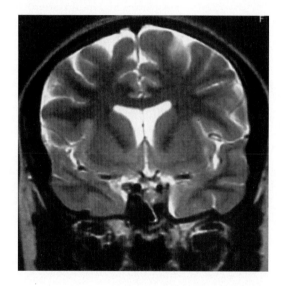

FIGURE 85.1C

CLINICAL HISTORY

A 26-year-old female with amenorrhea.

FINDINGS

Targeted noncontrast T1-weighted (Fig. 85.1A) images through the sella turcica demonstrate an ill-defined hypointense mass within the left side of the pituitary gland. There is a convex superior margin along the left side of the gland. Following intravenous contrast (Fig. 85.1B), the lesion remains hypointense. Tumor extends into the region of the left cavernous sinus with mild displacement of the cavernous carotid artery. There is no suprasellar extension. The optic chiasm is not displaced or compressed. Coronal T2-weighted acquisition (Fig. 85.1C) demonstrates a heterogeneous signal mass.

DIAGNOSIS

Pituitary microadenoma.

DISCUSSION

The presence of a focal lesion within the pituitary gland is the sine qua non of the diagnosis. However, not all focal lesions represent hormone-secreting microadenomas. It has been shown in previous autopsy studies, as well as clinical studies, that the incidence of incidental small pituitary lesions is on the order of 25% to 35% in normal individuals. These typically are Rathke's cleft cysts (20%), or nonfunctioning microadenomas in a smaller percentage of individuals. Thus finding a focal lesion is the radiographic criteria for the diagnosis, but hormonal criteria must be satisfied before the actual diagnosis can be made.

Pituitary microadenomas are hypercellular; thus the extracellular space between the individual cells is diminished, as compared with the loose stroma of the pituitary parenchyma itself. The lack of a blood-brain barrier means that contrast distributes quickly and diffusely through normal pituitary tissue but slowly into the packed extracellular space of a pituitary microneoplasm. This accounts for the relatively low signal intensity on contrast-enhanced MRI (and CT), but images need to be obtained quickly following contrast injection, as delayed imaging can allow the contrast to diffuse even into the tightly packed extracellular space of the tumor. Larger tumors are typically ones that enhance diffusely, given their abnormal blood supply as they grow.

The findings of asymmetric upward convexity of the gland and displacement of the stalk to the contralateral side are ancillary support for the diagnosis of pituitary tumor, even when a focal lesion cannot be identified. However, in and of themselves they are inadequate for the diagnosis of a lesion. Upward gland convexity can be normal. Normal gland height has been described as 12 to 13 mm, particularly in young women or pubertal adolescents.

SUGGESTED READINGS

Chong BW, Kucharczyk W, Singer W, et al. Pituitary gland MR: a comparative study of healthy volunteers and patients with microadenomas. *AJNR* 1994;15:675–679.

Davis PC, Hoffman JC Jr, Spencer T, et al. MR imaging of pituitary adenoma: CT, clinical, and surgical correlation. *AJNR* 1987;8:107–112.

Elster AD. Modern imaging of the pituitary. *Radiology* 1993;187:1–14.

Yuh WTC, Fisher DJ, Nguyen HD, et al. Sequential MR enhancement pattern in normal pituitary gland and in pituitary adenoma. *AJNR* 1994;15:101–108.

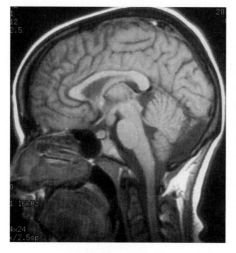

FIGURE 86.1A　　　　　　**FIGURE 86.1B**

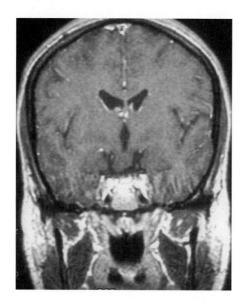

FIGURE 86.1C

CLINICAL HISTORY

A 20-year-old female patient who presented with agitation and headaches.

FINDINGS

There is a 1.5-cm mass in the suprasellar region that is isointense to brain on both T1- and T2-weighted sequences (Fig. 86.1A,B) and does not enhance with gadolinium (Fig. 86.1C).

DIAGNOSIS

Hamartoma of the tuber cinereum.

DISCUSSION

Also known as a hypothalamic hamartoma, this congenital malformation is composed of normal neuronal tissue arising from the posterior hypothalamus or mamillary bodies. Its incidence is greater in males than in females, and age at presentation is usually less than 2 years. Patients present with isosexual precocious puberty, neurodevelopmental delay, hyperactivity, and the often mentioned but rarely seen gelastic seizures.

On MRI this is usually seen as a well-defined round or oval mass projecting from the base of the brain into the suprasellar region. It is isointense on T1-weighted image and iso- to mildly hyperintense on T2-weighted image, basically following signal characteristics similar to gray matter.

Submitted by Sangita Patel, MD; William G. Bradley, MD, PhD, FACR (Senior Editor), Long Beach Memorial Medical Center, Long Beach, CA.

SUGGESTED READING

Boyko OB. Adult brain tumors. In: Stark DD, Bradley WG, eds. *Magnetic resonance imaging,* 3rd ed. St. Louis: Mosby, 1999:1231–1254.

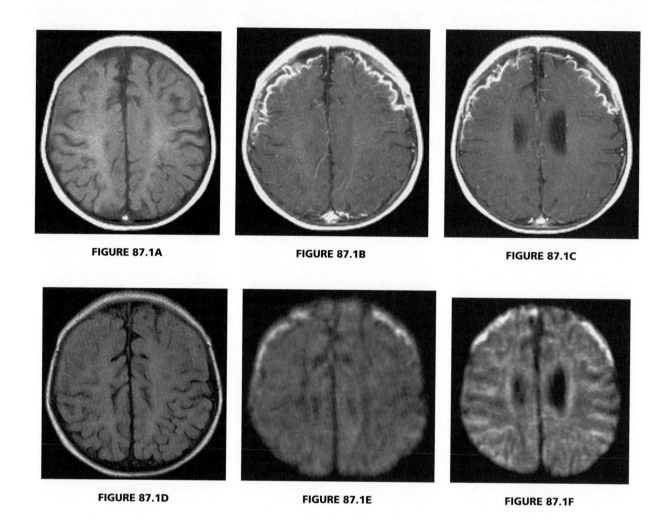

FIGURE 87.1A **FIGURE 87.1B** **FIGURE 87.1C**

FIGURE 87.1D **FIGURE 87.1E** **FIGURE 87.1F**

CLINICAL HISTORY

A young man with sepsis and altered mental status.

FINDINGS

Axial T1-weighted images demonstrate slight prominence of the lateral ventricles. Following contrast administration, irregular leptomeningeal enhancement over the frontal convexities is demonstrated (Fig. 87.1A–D), which is also bright on diffusion imaging (Fig. 87.1E,F).

DIAGNOSIS

Meningitis.

DISCUSSION

Meningitis is the most common infection of the central nervous system and involves the pia, arachnoid, and surrounding cerebrospinal fluid (CSF). Diagnosis is typically made on clinical grounds. Negative imaging studies do not exclude the diagnosis. Imaging is usually only obtained for suspected complications. Symptoms of meningitis include fever, headache, neck stiffness, change in mental status, and photophobia. Meningitis may occur from hematogenous spread or extension of contiguous infection such as otitis media or sinusitis. Most infections are bacterial (purulent) or viral (lymphocytic). The etiologic agent depends on the age and immune status of the patient. The most common infection in newborns is group B streptococcus. *Hemophilus influenzae* is seen commonly in young children, whereas older children and young adults are commonly affected by *Neisseria meningitides*. The most common agent in adults is *Streptococcus pneumoniae*. Tuberculosis, fungus, and sarcoid may cause chronic meningitis.

Nonenhanced CT examination is usually unremarkable. An early CT finding may be ventricular and subarachnoid space enlargement. Hydrocephalus may be obstructive or communicating, resulting from cellular debris or arachnoidal adhesions. Noncontrast CT may demonstrate sulcal or cisternal effacement from inflammatory exudate. Following contrast, abnormal leptomeningeal enhancement may be present that may extend deep into the sulci. Enhanced MR is more sensitive than enhanced CT. In severe chronic cases, the cerebrospinal fluid within the basal cisterns may be hyperintense on T1-weighted and proton-density-weighted sequences. Different etiologic agents may have different manifestations. A basilar cisternal predominance is present with tuberculosis and sarcoidosis. Meningeal sarcoid may also involve the hypothalamus, pituitary stalk, or optic chiasm, or produce thick meningeal plaques that mimic meningiomas.

The complications of meningitis are easily seen by MR. Complications include brain abscess, hydrocephalus, ventriculitis/ependymitis, or subdural empyemas or effusions (Fig. 87.1D). Purulent effusions may be longer on diffusion imaging (Fig. 87.1E,F). Arterial or venous infarctions may also occur secondary to perivascular inflammation and thrombosis.

Leptomeningeal enhancement is nonspecific. It may also be seen in leptomeningeal carcinomatosis, following surgery or shunt placement, or following subarachnoid hemorrhage.

Submitted by Stephanie Y. Chiu, MD; Peter Brotchie, MBBS, PhD; William G. Bradley, MD, PhD, FACR (Senior Editor), Long Beach Memorial Medical Center, Long Beach, CA.

SUGGESTED READINGS

Edelman RR, Hesselink JR, Zlatkin MB. *Clinical magnetic resonance imaging*, 2nd ed. Philadelphia: WB Saunders, 1996.
Osborn AG. *Diagnostic neuroradiology*. St. Louis: Mosby, 1994.

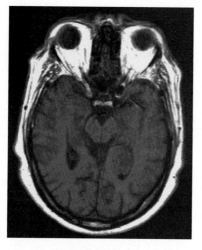

FIGURE 88.1A

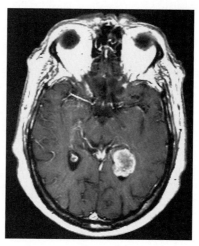

FIGURE 88.1B

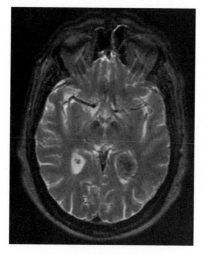

FIGURE 88.1C

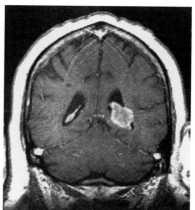

FIGURE 88.1D

CLINICAL HISTORY

A 55-year-old male with headaches.

FINDINGS

A mass is present within the atrium of the left lateral ventricle, demonstrating isointensity on T1 and heterogeneously low signal on T2-weighted relative to brain parenchyma (Fig. 88.1A,C). Fairly homogeneous intense enhancement is present (Fig. 88.1B,D). A corresponding CT examination demonstrated calcification.

DIAGNOSIS

Intraventricular meningioma.

DISCUSSION

Meningiomas are the most common extraaxial tumors and are usually benign. They most commonly occur in middle-aged adults and affect women more than men. The most common location is parasagittal. Other common locations are sphenoid wing, parasellar, and cerebellopontine angle. Intraventricular meningiomas only account for approximately 2% to 5% of all intracranial meningiomas.

Intraventricular meningiomas originate from either the tela choroidea or the choroid plexus. The most common location is the lateral ventricle, especially the left trigone. Less common is tumor in the third or fourth ventricles.

The appearance on MRI is similar to that of typical meningiomas. On nonenhanced MR, isointensity is the rule with occasional T1 and T2 hypointensity and T2 hyperintensity relative to brain parenchyma. Hypointensity on all pulse sequences can be seen with calcified lesions. There may be associated vasogenic edema in the adjacent brain due to cortical venous occlusion. Intense homogeneous enhancement is characteristic.

The main differential diagnosis of an intraventricular mass in an adult includes gliomas or metastases.

Submitted by Stephanie Y. Chiu, MD; Peter Brotchie, MBBS, PhD; William G. Bradley, MD, PhD, FACR (Senior Editor), Long Beach Memorial Medical Center, Long Beach, CA.

SUGGESTED READING

Buetow MP, Buetow PC, Smirniotopoulos JG, et al. Typical, atypical, and misleading features in meningioma. *Radiographics* 1991;11:1087–1106.

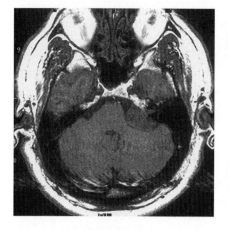

FIGURE 89.1A

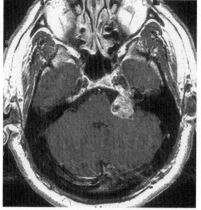

FIGURE 89.1B

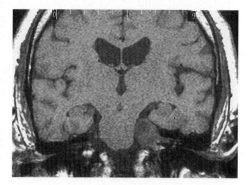

FIGURE 89.1C

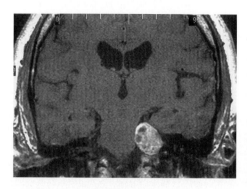

FIGURE 89.1D

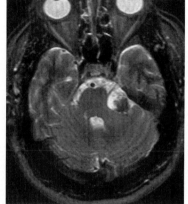

FIGURE 89.1E

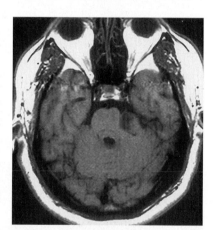

FIGURE 89.1F

CLINICAL HISTORY

A 59-year-old male who presents with left-sided hearing loss and vertigo.

FINDINGS

There is a 2.5-cm left cerebellopontine angle mass that demonstrates isointense signal on the precontrast T1-weighted images (Fig. 89.1A,C) and shows intense enhancement on the postcontrast images (Fig. 89.1B,D). There are subtle areas of cystic change, which are bright on T2-weighted images (Fig. 89.1E). Mild mass effect on the adjacent pons is noted (Fig. 89.1F).

DIAGNOSIS

Vestibular schwannoma.

DISCUSSION

Also referred to as an *acoustic schwannoma,* or neurilemoma, a vestibular schwannoma is an encapsulated neoplasm composed of proliferating fusiform Schwann cells with highly dense cellular regions (Antoni A) and loose areas with widely separated cells (Antoni B). Age at presentation ranges from 35 to 60 years with a predominance in females of 2:1. Bilateral schwannomas allow a presumptive diagnosis of NF 2. (Solitary schwannomas are associated with type 2 neurofibromatosis [NF 2] in only 5% to 25% of cases.) The patient presented with a history of progressive, unilateral sensorineural hearing loss, tinnitus, unsteadiness, vertigo, and ataxia.

This mass may arise within the internal auditory canal or in the cerebellopontine angle cistern at the porous acousticus. On MRI it is iso- to slightly hypointense on T1-weighted images relative to brain (Fig. 89.1A,C,F) and hyperintense on T2-weighted images (Fig 89.1E). Aside from areas of cystic degeneration (Antoni B), it enhances intensely and homogeneously after contrast administration. Associated findings include IAC erosion and enlargement, widening of the ipsilateral cerebellopontine (CP) angle cistern, shift of the fourth ventricle, and obstructive hydrocephalus (Fig. 89.1 C,D).

Submitted by Sangita Patel, MD; William G. Bradley, MD, PhD, FACR (Senior Editor), Long Beach Memorial Medical Center, Long Beach, CA.

SUGGESTED READING

Hirbawi IA, Hasso AN. Cranial nerves: normal anatomy and pathology. In: Stark DD, Bradley WG, eds. *Magnetic resonance imaging,* 3rd ed. St. Louis: Mosby, 1999:1209–1224.

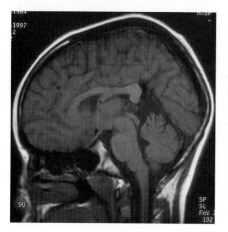

FIGURE 90.1A

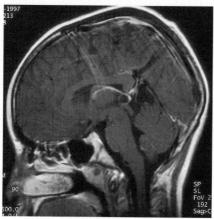

FIGURE 90.1B

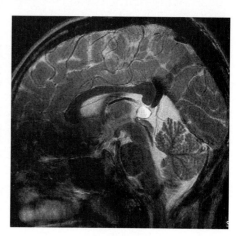

FIGURE 90.1C

CLINICAL HISTORY

A 45-year-old female with known breast carcinoma.

FINDINGS

There is a 1-cm rounded hypointense mass in the pineal region (Fig. 90.1A–C). This mass has a well-defined capsule and shows no enhancement on postcontrast images (Fig. 90.1B). It causes no mass effect on the adjacent brain parenchyma.

DIAGNOSIS

Pineal cyst.

DISCUSSION

Pineal cysts can be either developmental (persistence of an ependyma-lined diverticulum) or degenerative (cavitation within an area of gliosis). Although cysts may become symptomatic when large, they are usually seen incidentally on CT or MRI. They are not usually associated with Parinaud's syndrome nor do they cause hydrocephalus.

On MRI one sees a sharply marginated oval mass in the pineal region. They are slightly hyperintense to CSF on both T1-weighted and T2-weighted images. This reflects their higher protein content and the persistent phase coherence in cysts, which is absent in moving cerebrospinal fluid. One may also see slight contrast enhancement secondary to diffusion from peripheral, enhancing pineal tissue. The key differentiating point between these benign lesions and malignant pineal region tumors is the homogeneous signal intensity of the former (versus the heterogeneous signal of the latter).

Submitted by Sangita Patel, MD; William G. Bradley, MD, PhD, FACR (Senior Editor), Long Beach Memorial Medical Center, Long Beach, CA.

SUGGESTED READING

Jinkins JR, Xiong L, Reiter RJ. The midline pineal "eye": MR and CT characteristics of the pineal gland with and without benign cyst formation. *J Pineal Res* 1995;19:64–71.

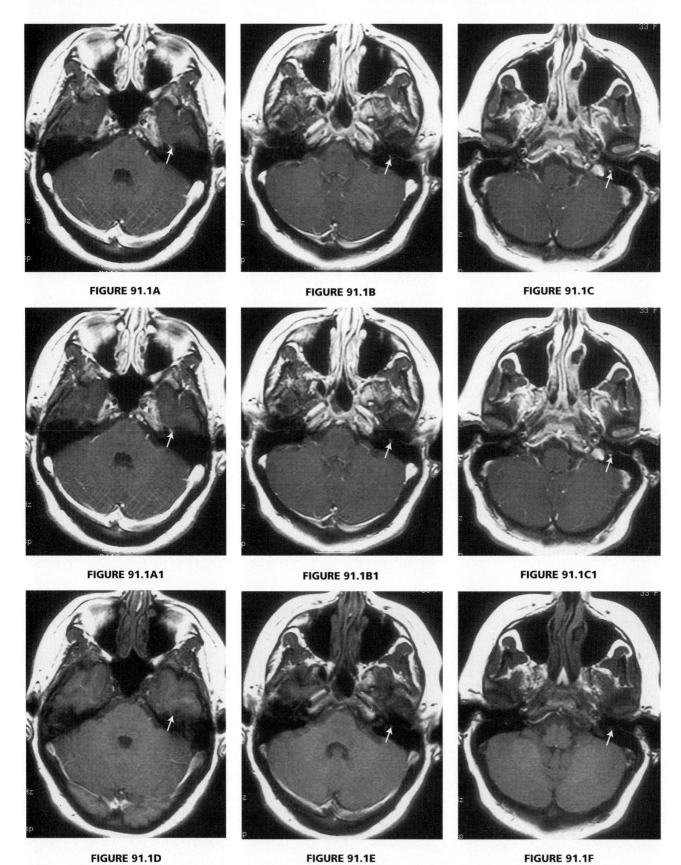

FIGURE 91.1A

FIGURE 91.1B

FIGURE 91.1C

FIGURE 91.1A1

FIGURE 91.1B1

FIGURE 91.1C1

FIGURE 91.1D

FIGURE 91.1E

FIGURE 91.1F

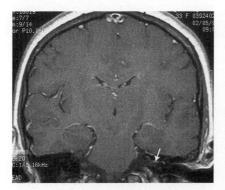
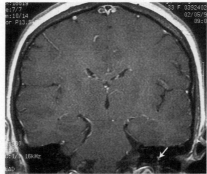
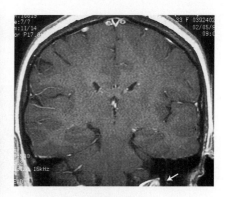

FIGURE 91.1G **FIGURE 91.1H** **FIGURE 91.1I**

CLINICAL HISTORY

A 37-year-old female patient with left-sided facial weakness and headaches.

FINDINGS

There is enhancement along the course of the labyrinthine, tympanic, and mastoid portions of the left facial nerve.

DIAGNOSIS

Bell's palsy.

DISCUSSION

Bell's palsy refers to an idiopathic facial nerve palsy that is the most common cause of lower motor neuron facial paralysis. It is thought to be caused by a viral infection with herpes simplex I and varicella zoster. The inflammation and hypervascularity lead to neural edema, which leads to nerve dysfunction. Onset of this disease can occur at any age and is usually self-limited, with resolution in 6 to 8 weeks.

Imaging is indicated in patients with atypical clinical findings or prolonged course (greater than 2 to 4 months) to exclude neoplastic or other infectious etiologies. Atypical findings include facial spasm, intense pain, or multiple cranial neuropathies.

Imaging diagnosis can be difficult, as the facial nerve can be seen to enhance mildly in normal patients due to associated vascular structures. However, classically, Bell's palsy produces marked enhancement of the facial nerve from the apex of the IAC (*arrows:* Fig. 91.1A,B,D,E,G) to the stylomastoid foramen (*arrows:* Fig. 91.1C,F,H,I). The resolution of the enhancement may lag behind clinical remission.

Submitted by Sangita Patel, MD; William G. Bradley, MD, PhD, FACR (Senior Editor), Long Beach Memorial Medical Center, Long Beach, CA.

SUGGESTED READING

Saatci I, Sahinturk F, Sennaroglu L, et al. MRI of the facial nerve in idiopathic facial palsy. *Eur Radiol* 1996;6:631–636.

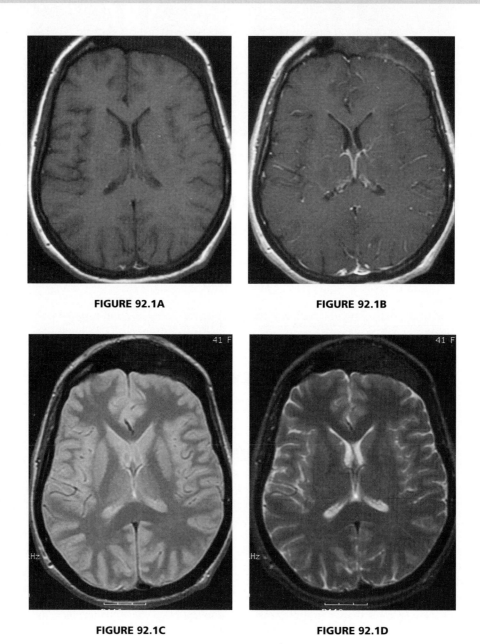

FIGURE 92.1A

FIGURE 92.1B

FIGURE 92.1C

FIGURE 92.1D

CLINICAL HISTORY

A 41-year-old female patient with headaches.

FINDINGS

There is expansion of the diploic space of the frontal bones more on the left than on the right, as well as involvement of the left anterior cranial fossa (Fig. 92.1A–D). There is heterogeneous signal enhancement with a "salt and pepper" appearance (Fig. 92.1B).

DIAGNOSIS

Fibrous dysplasia.

DISCUSSION

This is a benign fibroosseous developmental anomaly of mesenchymal bone. It can occur as a mono- or polyostotic process. In the craniofacial form (referred to as *leontiasis ossea*), frontal and sphenoid bone involvement are seen most commonly. Patients present with cranial asymmetry, facial deformity, exophthalmus, and visual impairment.

On imaging, one sees sclerotic lesions of the skull base, widened diploic spaces, and sparing of the inner table. (The differential diagnosis is Paget's disease, in which the inner table is involved.)

There can also be obliteration of the sphenoid and frontal sinuses, and cystic lesions of the calvarium.

Submitted by Sangita Patel, MD; William G. Bradley, MD, PhD, FACR (Senior Editor), Long Beach Memorial Medical Center, Long Beach, CA.

SUGGESTED READING

Jee WH, Choi KH, Choe BY, et al. Fibrous dysplasia: MR imaging characteristics with radiopathologic correlation. *AJR* 1996;167:1523–1527.

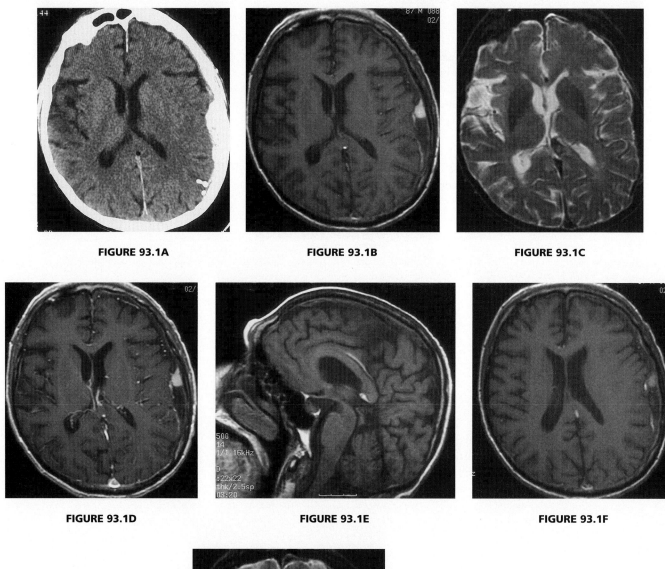

FIGURE 93.1A

FIGURE 93.1B

FIGURE 93.1C

FIGURE 93.1D

FIGURE 93.1E

FIGURE 93.1F

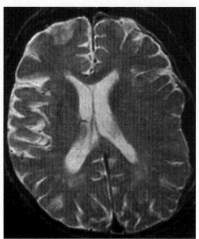

FIGURE 93.1G

CLINICAL HISTORY

An 88-year-old male with a history of dysphagia and weakness.

FINDINGS

There is a left convexity extraaxial fluid collection that is hyperdense on CT (Fig. 93.1A), primarily isointense on the T1-weighted (Fig. 93.1B,F) images and hypointense on the T2-weighted images (Fig. 93.1C,G). There are also areas of hyperintense signal on the T1-weighted images in the extraaxial compartment, which do not enhance (Fig. 93.1D) and next to the corpus callosum (Fig. 93.1E).

DIAGNOSIS

Subdural hematoma and incidental callosal lipoma.

DISCUSSION

Subdural hematoma (SDH) occurs as a result of tears of bridging veins and attached dural sinuses. Hemorrhage occurs into the potential space between the arachnoid membrane and the dura mater. It freely extends across suture lines, limited only by the falx in the interhemispheric fissure and the tentorium. There is no consistent relationship to skull fractures.

SDH occurs in 5% of head trauma patients and in 65% of trauma patients with prolonged interruption of consciousness. It occurs predominantly in infants and the elderly.

The appearance of the hemorrhage depends on the stage of blood products. Acute blood (intracellular deoxyhemoglobin) is isointense on T1-weighted and hypointense on T2-weighted images. Late subacute hemorrhage (extracellular methemoglobin) appears hyperintense on both T1- and T2-weighted images. These are the main components of this SDH. Chronic subdural collections are hyperintense to cerebrospinal fluid on T1-, proton-density-weighted, and FLAIR weighted images (seen in the middle of the SDH). Both acute and subacute or chronic hemorrhage are seen with recurrent bleeding (as in this case).

Also seen is a callosal lipoma. This is a congenital pericallosal tumor. When they are located anteriorly and are cylindrical, these can be associated with anomalies of the corpus callosum, interhemispheric arachnoid cysts, frontal bone defects, encephaloceles, and cutaneous lipomas. Patients may be symptomatic, with seizure disorders or mental retardation. When they are located posteriorly and they are curvilinear (as in this case), they are usually asymptomatic.

MRI shows a hyperintense midline mass superior to the corpus callosum on T1-weighted images (Fig. 93.1E,F) that turns dark on the conventional (as opposed to fast) T2-weighted spin-echo image (Fig. 93.1G).

Submitted by Sangita Patel, MD; William G. Bradley, MD, PhD, FACR (Senior Editor), Long Beach Memorial Medical Center, Long Beach, CA.

SUGGESTED READINGS

Bradley WG. Hemorrhage. In: Stark DD, Bradley WG, eds. *Magnetic resonance imaging,* 3rd ed. St. Louis: Mosby, 1999:1329–1346.

Evans SJJ, Gean D. Craniocerebral trauma. In: Stark DD, Bradley WG, eds. *Magnetic resonance imaging,* 3rd ed. St. Louis: Mosby, 1999:1347–1360.

Tart RP, Quisling RG. Curvilinear and tubulonodular varieties of lipoma of the corpus callosum: an MR and CT study. *JCAT* 1991;(15):805–810.

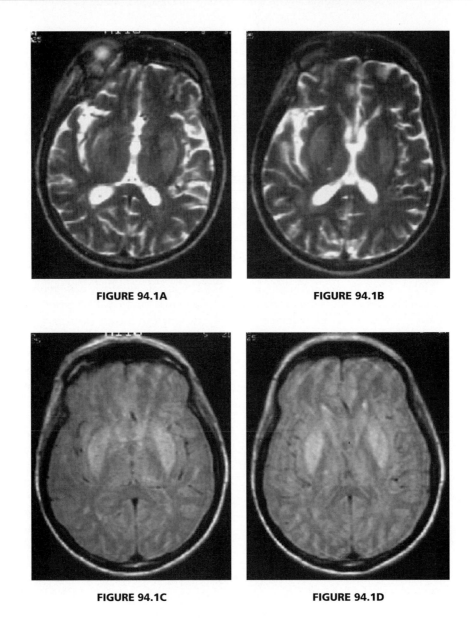

FIGURE 94.1A

FIGURE 94.1B

FIGURE 94.1C

FIGURE 94.1D

CLINICAL HISTORY

A 54-year-old male with progressive dementia and extrapyramidal symptoms.

FINDINGS

Bilateral increased signal intensity is present in both thalami and lentiform nuclei on T2- (Fig. 94.1A,B) and proton-density-weighted images (Fig. 94.1C,D). No mass effect or necrosis is seen. No enhancement was evident after giving gadolinium.

DIAGNOSIS

Creutzfeldt-Jakob disease.

DISCUSSION

Creutzfeldt-Jakob disease is a rare, fatal brain disorder. It affects about one person in a million. Typically, onset of symptoms occurs at about age 60, with 90% fatality after 1 year. The disease is believed to be caused by a protein called a *prion*. The causative agent differs from any other recognized organism in that it does not contain any DNA or RNA and is not killed by the usual sterilization methods. In the early stages of the disease, patients may have failing memory, behavioral changes, lack of coordination, and visual disturbances. As the illness progresses, mental deterioration becomes more pronounced, with involuntary movements, blindness, weakness of extremities, and eventually coma.

On MRI, T2-weighted images reveal bilateral increased signal intensity in the putamen, globus pallidus, caudate nucleus, and thalamus, with no mass effect or necrosis. The T1-weighted images are usually unremarkable and do not show enhancement with gadolinium.

Submitted by Sattam Lingawi, MB, ChB; Peter Brotchie, MBBS, PhD; William G. Bradley, MD, PhD, FACR (Senior Editor), Long Beach Memorial Medical Center, Long Beach, CA.

SUGGESTED READING

Finkenstaedt M, Szudra A, Zerr I, et al. MR imaging of Creutzfeldt-Jakob disease. *Radiology* 1996;199:793–798.

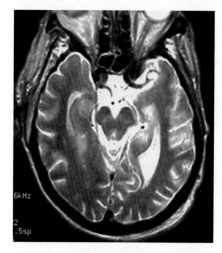

FIGURE 95.1A

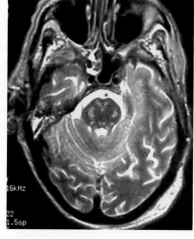

FIGURE 95.1B

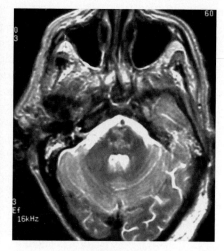

FIGURE 95.1C

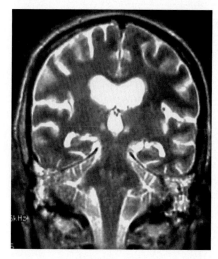

FIGURE 95.1D

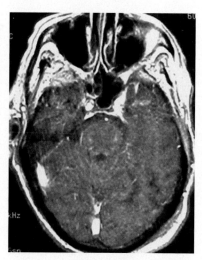

FIGURE 95.1E

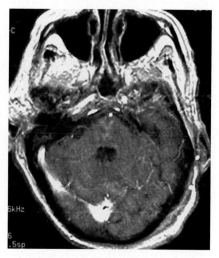

FIGURE 95.1F

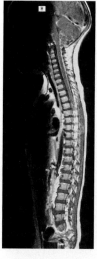

FIGURE 95.1G

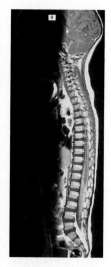

FIGURE 95.1H

CLINICAL HISTORY

A 60-year-old male with history of cirrhosis who has received a liver transplant. The patient has persistent encephalopathy.

FINDINGS

Axial and coronal T2-weighted images (Fig. 95.1A–D) demonstrate symmetrically abnormal high signal within the thalami, base of Pons, medulla, and periaqueductal gray matter. Postcontrast T1-weighted images (Fig. 95.1E, F) show patchy enhancement of these lesions.

DIAGNOSIS

Pontine and extrapontine osmotic myelinolysis (OM).

DISCUSSION

OM is a toxic demyelinating disease that typically occurs in alcoholic, malnourished, and chronically debilitated patients with severe electrolyte disturbances. Most cases are associated with chronic alcoholism in the setting of rapid correction of hyponatremia. The symptoms of OM are quadraparesis, pseudobulbar palsy, and decreased level of consciousness, often resulting in coma and/or death.

Pathologically, OM is characterized by myelin loss with relative sparing of the neuron. The central pons is the most common site, hence the term *central pontine myelinolysis* (CPM) (see Vol. 2, Case 20). OM also occurs in extrapontine locations (50% of cases), such as putamina, caudate nuclei, midbrain, thalami, and subcortical white matter (see in this case).

Nonenhanced CT scans are frequently normal or show subtle hypodensity in the affected areas. On MRI, OM is typically hypointense on T1-weighted images and hyperintense on T2-weighted scans. The characteristic appearance of CPM on PD- and T2-weighted images is a central trian-gular region of hyperintense signal, simulating a "trefoil" hat (see Case 20). This pattern reflects the propensity of OM to most severely affect the central transverse fibers, with characteristic sparing of the descending corticospinal tracts, the peripheral pial and ventricular surface rim of tissue. Enhancement is uncommon but can occur, most frequently at the periphery of the lesion (shown in this case).

Extrapontine myelinolysis can occur without the presence of pontine disease. Temporal studies have shown MRI findings to lag behind clinical signs of improvement. Lesions may not completely resolve despite clinical recovery.

The differential diagnosis for nonenhancing high signal in the pons includes infarct, glioma, multiple sclerosis, progressive multifocal leukoencephalopathy, rhomben-cephalitis, and radiation or chemotherapy change. If there is abnormal signal within the basal ganglia as well, the findings are more specific for osmotic myelinolysis. Differential diagnosis would still include hypoxia, Leigh disease (see Vol. I, Case 90), and Wilson disease.

SUGGESTED READINGS

Hadfield MG, Kubal WS. Extrapontine myelinolysis of the basal ganglia without central pontine myelinolysis. *Clin Neuropathol* 1996;15:96–100.

Huin E, Tan KP. CT and MR findings in central pontine and extrapontine myelinolysis—a study of two patients. *Singapore Med J* 1996;37:622–666.

Laubenberger J, Schneider B, Ansorge O, et al. Central pontine myelinolysis: clinical presentation and radiologic findings. *Eur Radiol* 1996;6:177–183.

Miller GM, Baker HL Jr, Okozaki H, et al. Central pontine myelinolysis and its imitators: MR findings. *Radiology* 1988;168:795–802.

Valk J, van der Knaap MS. Toxic encephalopathy. *AJNR* 1992;13:747–760.

Yuh WT, Simonson TM, D'Alessandro MP, et al. Temporal changes of MR findings in central pontine myelinolysis. *AJNR* 1995;16[Suppl]:975–977.

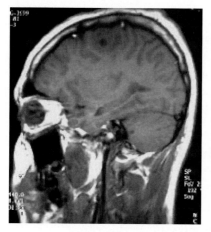

FIGURE 96.1A

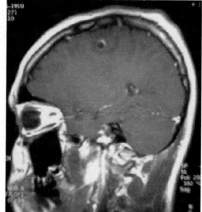

FIGURE 96.1B

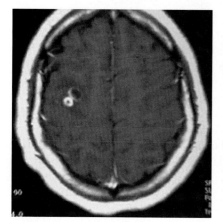

FIGURE 96.1C

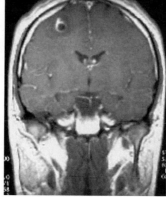

FIGURE 96.1D

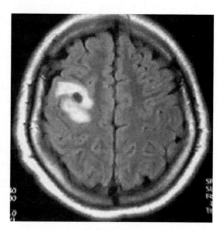

FIGURE 96.1E

CLINICAL HISTORY

A 14-year-old male with new onset of seizures.

FINDINGS

Two small cystic lesions with ring enhancement are evident in the right frontal lobe on the T1-weighted images (Fig. 96.1A–D). Mild surrounding vasogenic edema is seen on the FLAIR image (Fig. 96.1E).

DIAGNOSIS

Cysticercosis.

DISCUSSION

Neurocysticercosis is an infestation of the central nervous system by larvae of *Taenia solium,* the pork tapeworm. The parasite is ingested when eating undercooked pork or contaminated food. The larvae hatch in the intestine and are distributed systemically, with a predilection for the muscles and brain.

Patients are usually asymptomatic until the larvae die. The larval death incites an intense host reaction resulting in extensive cerebral edema. The most common presenting symptom is seizures. Patients may also present with symptoms of basal meningitis, intracranial hypertension, arach-noiditis, and dementia. Intraventricular cysticercosis is potentially life threatening because of cerebrospinal fluid dissemination and acute obstructive hydrocephalus. The racemose form of the infestation is characterized by multilocular, nonviable cysts of variable sizes that lack the parasitic scolex, most commonly located in the basal cisterns.

On MRI, parenchymal cysticercosis is usually hypointense on T1- and hyperintense on T2-weighted images with a scolex in the cystic component of the parasite. Surrounding edema is often present. Old lesions frequently calcify.

Submitted by Sattam Lingawi, MB, ChB; Peter Brotchie, MBBS, PhD; William G. Bradley, MD, PhD, FACR (Senior Editor), Long Beach Memorial Medical Center, Long Beach, CA.

SUGGESTED READING

Suss RA, Maravilla KR, Thompson J. MR imaging of intracranial cysticercosis: comparison with CT and anatomopathologic features. *AJNR* 1986;7:235–242.

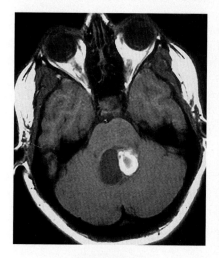

FIGURE 97.1A

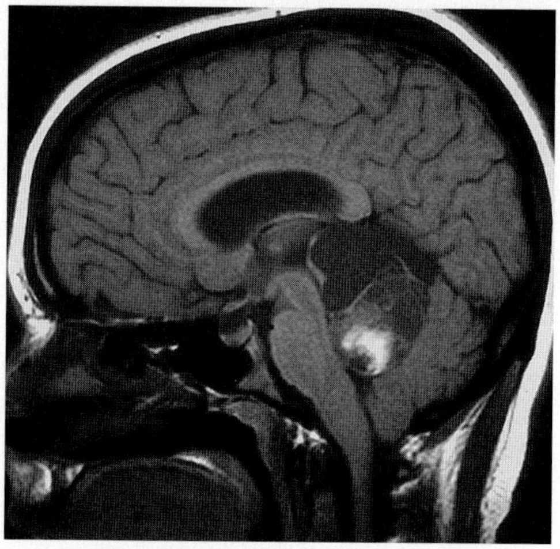

FIGURE 97.1B

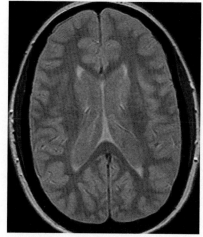

FIGURE 97.1C

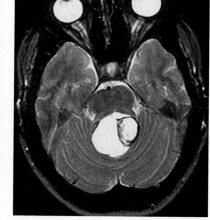

FIGURE 97.1D

CLINICAL HISTORY

A 23-year-old female with increasing headaches.

FINDINGS

There is a large, cystic mass with an enhancing nodule in the fourth ventricle (Fig. 97.1A,B) causing obstructive hydrocephalus (Fig.97.1C). On T2-weighted images (Fig. 97.1D), there is evidence of hemosiderin staining, indicating that there has been prior bleeding.

DIAGNOSIS

Fourth ventricular ependymoma.

DISCUSSION

There are three common types of gliomas in the brain: astrocytomas, oligodendrogliomas, and ependymomas. The latter tend to be more common in the fourth ventricle in both children and adults but can also occur in the lateral ventricles in children. Because the ependyma is very vascular, these tumors tend to enhance with gadolinium and to bleed—which accounts for the hemosiderin staining (Fig. 97.1D). Notice that the tumor cyst has higher intensity than that of cerebrospinal fluid (CSF). This reflects the higher protein content of the tumor cyst with consequent shortening of the T1 relaxation time (Fig. 97.1B). In this way, tumor cysts can always be distinguished from uncomplicated arachnoid cysts, which contain CSF. Tumors located in strategic positions within the ventricular system—like the fourth ventricle or the aqueduct—often present as a result of obstructive hydrocephalus rather than local invasion—as was the case here. A smooth border of high signal intensity surrounding the lateral ventricles on the proton-density-weighted image is indicative of elevated intracranial pressure with secondary transependymal resorption of CSF or "interstitial edema." Over time, the ventricles will expand until the mean intraventricular pressure is normal. This process is called *compensation*. With compensation, the interstitial edema gradually resorbs and the smooth border of high signal intensity goes away (Fig. 97.1C).

Submitted by William G. Bradley, MD, PhD, FACR (Senior Editor) Long Beach Memorial Medical Center, Long Beach, CA.

SUGGESTED READINGS

Boyko OB. Adult brain tumors. In: Stark DD, Bradley WG, eds. *Magnetic resonance imaging,* 3rd ed. St. Louis: Mosby, 1999:1231–1254.

Bradley WG, Quencer RM. Hydrocephalus and cerebrospinal fluid flow. In: Stark DD, Bradley WG, eds. *Magnetic resonance imaging,* 3rd ed. St. Louis: Mosby, 1999:1483–1508.

Lefton DR, Pinto RS, Martin SW. MRI features of intracranial and spinal ependymomas. *Pediatr Neurosurg* 1998;28:97–105.

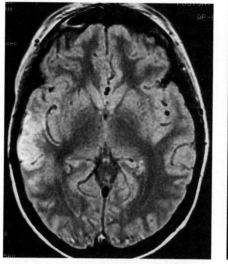

FIGURE 98.1A

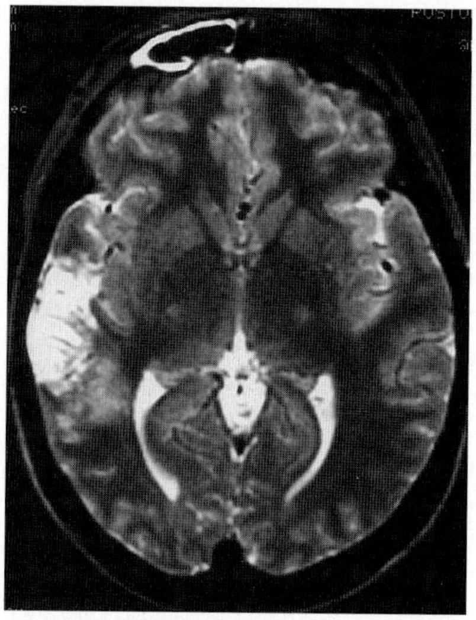

FIGURE 98.1B

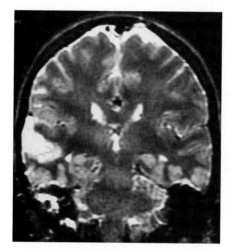

FIGURE 98.1C

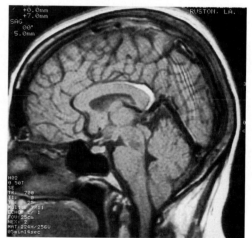

FIGURE 98.1D

CLINICAL HISTORY

A 35-year-old female with head trauma 4 months previously.

FINDINGS

Right temporal encephalomalacia is noted on the proton-density- and T2-weighted axial and coronal views (Fig. 98.1A–C). The sagittal T1-weighted image (Fig. 98.1D) demonstrates curvilinear high signal surrounding the splenium of the corpus callosum, which appears dark on the conventional T2-weighted coronal image (Fig. 98.1C).

DIAGNOSIS

(1) Posttraumatic right temporal encephalomalacia. (2) Incidental lipoma of the corpus callosum.

DISCUSSION

Encephalomalacia can be subdivided into microcystic and macrocystic forms. Microcystic encephalomalacia consists of multiple small cysts with sufficient aggregate surface area to bind water in hydration layers, shortening the T1 (similar to a proteinaceous solution). This is the reason that microcystic encephalomalacia (or *gliosis*) is relatively bright on a proton-density-weighted or FLAIR image. Macrocystic encephalomalacia represents much larger cysts without sufficient surface area to cause significant T1 shortening. Macrocystic encephalomalacia therefore appears to have the same intensity as bulk phase water (e.g., cerebrospinal fluid). Both types of encephalomalacia are noted here following evacuation of a hematoma following head trauma.

Lipomas of the corpus callosum are generally incidental findings of no clinical significance—unless they are misinterpreted as subacute, subdural hematomas in patients with previous head trauma. The fat signal in the callosal lipoma tracks with that of subcutaneous fat (i.e., bright on a T1-weighted image and dark on a T2-weighted conventional spin-echo image, but relatively bright on a T2-weighted fast spin-echo image).

Submitted by William G. Bradley, MD, PhD, FACR (Senior Editor) Long Beach Memorial Medical Center, Long Beach, CA.

SUGGESTED READINGS

Bradley WG. Pathophysiologic correlates of signal alteration. In: Brant-Zawadzki M, Norman D, eds. *Magnetic resonance in the central nervous system.* New York: Raven Press, 1986.
Suzuki M, Takashima T, Kadoya M, et al. Pericallosal lipomas: MR features. *JCAT* 1991;15:207–209.

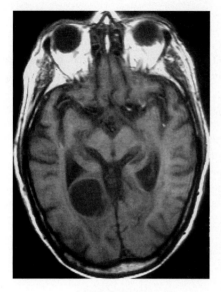

FIGURE 99.1A

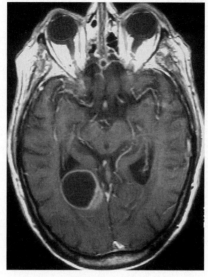

FIGURE 99.1B

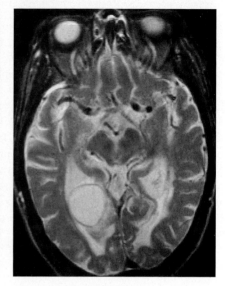

FIGURE 99.1C

CLINICAL HISTORY

An 86-year-old male patient with stuttering onset of left homonymous hemianopsia, rule out CVA.

FINDINGS

There is a 3-cm mass in the right occipital lobe. It demonstrates intense peripheral enhancement with an irregular soft tissue component medially (Fig. 99.1A,B). There is moderate surrounding edema (Fig. 99.1C).

DIAGNOSIS

Parenchymal metastasis.

DISCUSSION

The most common primary tumors to metastasize to the brain include bronchial carcinoma, breast, GI-tract tumors, renal cell carcinoma, and melanoma. They usually involve the corticomedullary junction of the brain (80%) or the leptomeninges (20%). The primary differential diagnoses of a mass in a patient more than 60 years old is an isolated metastasis. In a patient less than 60 years of age, it is a primary glioma. Twenty percent to 40% of metastases are isolated when they first present.

The usual presentation for parenchymal metastasis is multiple lesions of varying sizes with associated mass effect and enhancement on postcontrast images. On MRI one sees homogeneous or nodular peripheral enhancement on postcontrast images, and extensive edema on T2-weighted images. Leptomeningeal metastases demonstrate enhancement extending from the cortical surface into the sulci, best seen on postcontrast FLAIR images.

Submitted by Sangita Patel, MD; William G. Bradley, MD, PhD, FACR (Senior Editor), Long Beach Memorial Medical Center, Long Beach, CA.

SUGGESTED READING

Boyko OB. Adult brain tumors. In: Stark DD, Bradley WG, eds. *Magnetic resonance imaging,* 3rd ed. St. Louis: Mosby, 1999:1231–1254.

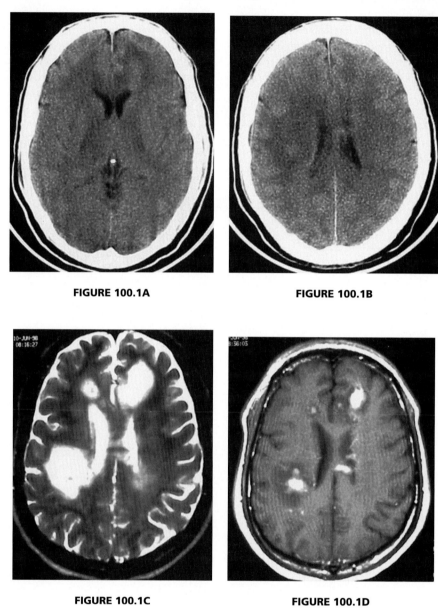

FIGURE 100.1A

FIGURE 100.1B

FIGURE 100.1C

FIGURE 100.1D

CASE 100A

CLINICAL HISTORY

Right leg weakness with left hand pain and weakness.

FINDINGS

Axial noncontrast CT acquisition (Fig. 100.1A,B) shows subtle hyperdense lesions within the left frontal and right parietal lobes with surrounding vasogenic edema. Axial T2-weighted and postcontrast T1-weighted images (Fig. 100.1B–D) demonstrate large rounded enhancing lesions within both frontal lobes and the right parietal lobe. Smaller enhancing lesions are seen within the corpus callosum to the left of midline.

DIAGNOSIS

Primary central nervous system lymphoma.

CASE 100B

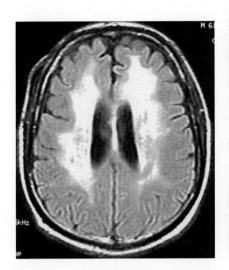 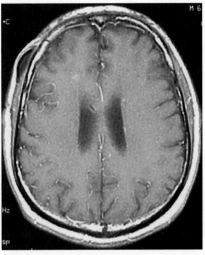

FIGURE 100.1E   **FIGURE 100.1F**

CLINICAL HISTORY

Three months after radiation therapy and intrathecal methotrexate the same patient presented with mental status change.

FINDINGS

Axial FLAIR acquisition (Fig. 100.1E) shows confluent abnormal high signal throughout the deep white matter of both hemispheres. The large spherical lesions seen on the previous study are no longer identified. Following contrast (Fig. 100.1F) there is only faint residual enhancement of the right frontal lobe lesion. Note the omaya reservoir within the scalp in the right frontal region with associated ventricular catheter.

DIAGNOSIS

Disseminated necrotizing leukoencephalopathy.

DISCUSSION

Neurotoxicity is a well-known complication of radiation and chemotherapy treatment. Chemotherapeutic agents known to cause leukoencephalopathy include cyclosporin A, methotrexate, cytarabine, cisplatin, and 5-fluorouracil.

Diffuse necrotizing leukoencephalopathy (DNL) is a condition typically seen in patients receiving a combination of intrathecal methotrexate, intravenous methotrexate, and cerebral irradiation. Patients typically present with rapid clinical deterioration several months after treatment is initiated, including cognitive dysfunction, ataxia, and/or dementia. The combination of chemotherapy and adjuvant radiotherapy causes a necrotizing angiitis, which results in multifocal coagulative necrosis of white matter, myelin degeneration, swollen axons, calcification, and enlarged reactive astrocytes.

At imaging, DNL appears as confluent, symmetric deep white matter hypodensity on CT with corresponding high signal on T2-weighted MR images (as demonstrated in this case). The central and periventricular white matter is primarily involved with relative sparing of the subcortical U fibers. The corpus callosum is usually not involved. Small multifocal regions of white matter enhancement have been reported. Findings may be reversible or progressive. If the patient survives, the necrotic areas retract and white matter atrophy ensues.

SUGGESTED READINGS

Asato R, Akiyama Y, Ito M, et al. Nuclear magnetic resonance abnormalities of the cerebral white matter in children with acute lymphoblastic leukemia and malignant lymphoma during and after central nervous system prophylactic treatment with intrathecal methotrexate. *Cancer* 1992;70:1997–2004.

Kieme-Guibert F, Napolitano M, Delattre JY. Neurologic complications of radiation therapy and chemotherapy. *J Neurol* 1998;245:695–708.

Laxmi SN, Takahashi S, Matsumoto K, et al. Treatment related disseminated necrotizing leukoencephalopathy with characteristic contrast enhancement of the white matter. *Radiat Med* 1996;14:303–307.

Sakamaki H, Onozowa Y, Yano Y, et al. Disseminated necrotizing leukoencephalopathy following irradiation and methotrexate therapy for central nervous system infiltration of leukemia and lymphoma. *Radiat Med* 1993;11:146–153.

Valk PE, Dillon WP. Radiation injury of the brain. *AJNR* 1991;12:45–62.

SUBJECT INDEX

thrombosis, sagittal sinus, 43–44
Meningitis, 182–183
    basal, cysticercosis, 201
    cryptococcal, 124–125
Meningoencephalitis, herpes, 15
Meninx primitiva, development of, 127
Mental confusion. *See also* Mental status
    Creutzfeldt-Jakob disease, 197
    cysticercosis, 201
    Hallervorden-Spatz disease, 115
    Huntington's disease, 39
    progressive, Creutzfeldt-Jakob disease,
        196
    subdural hematoma, 172
    vertigo and, 4
    Wernicke encephalopathy, 136, 137
Mental retardation, corpus callosum,
        agenesis of, 31
Mental status
    altered, 63
        cerebral venous thrombosis, 155
        meningitis, 182
    systemic lupus erythematosus, 98
Mesial temporal sclerosis, 139
Metabolic alteration, basal ganglia, related to
        chronic liver disease, 164–165
Methotrexate
    intrathecal, central nervous system
        lymphoma, 209
    leukoencephalopathy from, 209
Microadenoma, pituitary, 29, 178–179
    amenorrhea, 178
Microscopic encephalomalacia, macrocystic
        encephalomalacia, distinguished,
        205
Migraine, 9
    moyamoya disease, 52
Miosis, medullary infarct and, 10
Morning headache, fourth ventricular
        ependymoma, 146
Motor neuron, facial paralysis, 191
Movement, choreaform, Huntington's
        disease, 38
Moyamoya disease, 52–53
MS. *See* Multiple sclerosis
MTS. *See* Mesial temporal sclerosis
"Mulberry" lesions, cavernous hemangioma,
        77
Multiple meningioma, in neurofibromatosis
        type II, 109
Multiple sclerosis, 105
    basilar artery ectasia, 73
    migraine and, 9
    tumefactive, 19, 93–94
Mycobacterium tuberculosis, 23
Myelinolysis, pontine, 40–41, 199

N

Nausea
    with central nervous system hydatid
        disease, 129

with cerebral venous thrombosis, 155
with headache, 2
with hemorrhagic metastases, melanoma,
        131
Neck, stiff, with headache, 2
Necrotizing granulomatous vasculitis,
        104–105
Necrotizing leukoencephalopathy, 209
Neisseria meningitides, meningitis, 183
Neuralgia, trigeminal, 80
    basilar artery ectasia, 73
Neurilemoma, acoustic, 187
Neuritis, optic, multiple sclerosis, 18
Neurocysticercosis, 201
Neurocytoma, central, 161
Neurodevelopmental delay, hamartoma of
        tuber cinereum, 181
Neuroectodermal tumor, dysembryoplastic,
        74
Neuroendocrine symptoms, hemorrhagic
        pituitary adenoma, 67
Neuroepithelial tumor, dysembryoplastic,
        148–149
Neurofibromatosis type II, multiple
        meningioma in, 109
Neuropathy, cranial
    brainstem astrocytoma, 32
    headache and, 2
Neurotoxicity, as complication of radiation,
        chemotherapy treatment, 209
Normal pressure hydrocephalus, 7
NPH. *See* Normal pressure hydrocephalus
Numbness
    facial
        lateral medullary infarct, 168
        Wallenberg's syndrome, 11
    lateral medullary infarct, 168
    medullary infarct and, 10

O

Obstructive hydrocephalus, 153
Ocular muscle, paralysis of, Wernicke
        encephalopathy, 137
Oligodendroglioma, intraventricular, 161
Ophthalmoplegia, Wernicke
        encephalopathy, 137
Optic nerve atrophy, Hallervorden-Spatz
        disease, 115
Optic neuritis, multiple sclerosis, 18
Oral contraceptives, cerebral venous
        thrombosis, 155
Osmotic myelinolysis, 40–41
    pontine, 199
Osteochondroma
    arising from left petrous apex, 17
Ovarian metastases, to brain, 63–64

P

Paget's disease, 193
Palsy
    central pontine myelinolysis, 41

cranial nerve, central nervous system
        hydatid disease, 129
    facial, dural sinus thrombosis and, 13
    facial nerve, 191
    pseudobulbar, pontine osmotic
        myelinolysis, 199
    sixth nerve, brainstem astrocytoma, 33
Papilledema, central nervous system hydatid
        disease, 129
Parafalcine meningioma, 109
Paralysis, ocular muscle, Wernicke
        encephalopathy, 137
Parenchymal hematoma, epidural, parietal
        fracture, 79
Parenchymal hemorrhage, dural sinus
        thrombosis with, 13
Parenchymal metastasis, 162–163, 206–207
Parenchymal TB infection, tuberculoma, 23
Paresis, of upward gaze, 111
Paresthesias, necrotizing granulomatous
        vasculitis, 104
Parietal fracture, with epidural, parenchymal
        hematoma, 79
Parinaud's syndrome, 111, 189
    from pineal cysts, 177
Partial complex seizures
    dysembryoplastic neuroepithelial tumor,
        148
    ganglioglioma, 166
Pericallosal lipoma, corpus callosum
        dysgenesis with, 127
Perilesional edema, with metastases, 63
Periventricular abnormalities, migraine and,
        9
Personality change, central nervous system
        lymphoma, 122
Personality disorder, Huntington's disease,
        39
Petrous apex, osteochondroma arising from,
        17
Pigment, iron, deposition of, within
        extrapyramidal nuclei, 115
Pilocytic astrocytoma, 91
    juvenile, 167
Pineal gland
    cyst, 176–177, 188–189
    neoplasm, 111
    signal intensity, 188
Pineocytoma, 110–111
Pituitary dwarfism, short statute, 159
Pituitary gland
    adenohypophysis, 29
    adenoma, hemorrhagic, 67
    macroadenoma, 48–49, 112–113
    microadenoma, 29, 178–179
    posterior, ectopic, 158–159
Planum sphenoidal meningioma, 135
Pleomorphic xanthoastrocytoma, 167
Poisoning
    carbon monoxide, anoxia due to, 65

Upward gaze, paresis of, 111
Urinary incontinence, 7

V

Vaccination, encephalomyelitis triggered by, 151
Varicella zoster, facial paralysis, 191
Vascular malformation, intraparenchymal hemorrhage, 155
Vasculitis
  granulomatous, necrotizing, 104–105
  migraine and, 9
Vasogenic edema, reversible, 89
Venous angioma, cavernous hemangioma with, 141
Venous infarction
  dural sinus thrombosis with secondary parenchymal hemorrhage, 13
  hemorrhagic, superior sagittal sinus thrombosis, 155–156
  intraparenchymal hemorrhage, 155
Ventricular ependymoma, 147
  fourth, 202–203
Ventriculitis, meningitis, 183
Ventriculoperitoneal shunt
  communicating hydrocephalus, following subarachnoid hemorrhage, 36
  normal pressure hydrocephalus, 7
Vertigo
  brainstem astrocytoma, 33
  Hallervorden-Spatz disease, 115

normal pressure hydrocephalus, 7
  pineocytoma, 110
  superficial siderosis and, 4
  vestibular schwannoma, 186, 187
Vestibular schwannoma, 186–187
Viral infection
  encephalomyelitis triggered by, 151
  facial paralysis, 191
  herpes encephalitis, 15
Visual disturbance
  Creutzfeldt-Jakob disease, 197
  cysticercosis, 20
  fibrous dysplasia, 193
  meningioma with destruction of calvarium, 46
  pineocytoma, 110
  pituitary macroadenoma, 112
  tectal glioma with benign meningeal fibrosis, 116
  tuberculoma, 22
Visual field defects, hemorrhagic pituitary adenoma, 67
Voice, sensation of hearing own, with headache, 2
Voluntary movements, slowing of, Hallervorden-Spatz disease, 115
Vomiting
  with central nervous system hydatid disease, 129
  with cerebral venous thrombosis, 155
  with headache, 2

hemorrhagic metastases, melanoma, 131
Von-Hippel Lindau disease, difficulty walking, 50

W

Walking, difficulty. *See also* Gait disturbance
  Von-Hippel Lindau disease, 50
Wallenberg's syndrome, 169
  facial numbness, 11
Wallerian degeneration, axonal injury, diffuse, 35
Weakness
  central nervous system lymphoma, 208
  of extremities, Creutzfeldt-Jakob disease, 197
  leg, parafalcine meningioma, 108
  moyamoya disease, 52
  necrotizing granulomatous vasculitis, 104
  subdural hematoma, 194
  superior sagittal sinus thrombosis with hemorrhagic venous infarction, 154
  tuberculoma, 22
  tumefactive multiple sclerosis, 92
Wernicke encephalopathy, 137
Wernicke-Korsakoff syndrome, 137
White matter ischemia, normal pressure hydrocephalus, 7
Wilson disease, 199

X

Xanthoastrocytoma, pleomorphic, 167